Healthy Foods

and

Spiritual Nutrition

handbook

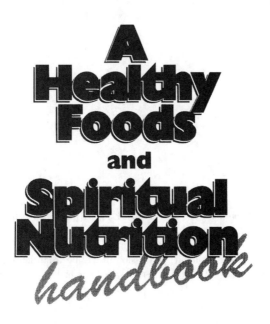

A Healthy Foods and Spiritual Nutrition handbook

A comprehensive guide to good food and a healthy lifestyle

Keith Wright

EWORLD INC.

1200 Jefferson Avenue
Buffalo, NY 14208

formerly ISBN: 0-9625285-0-7

COVER DESIGN: *EWorld Inc.*
COVER ILLUSTRATION: *Andre Harris*
ISBN 978-1-61759-007-8

Formally published by
A&B Publishers Group
Brooklyn, New York
ISBN 1-881316-97-1

CIP Data

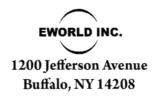

EWORLD INC.
1200 Jefferson Avenue
Buffalo, NY 14208

10 11 12   5 4 3 2 1

Dedication

This book is dedicated to my mother, the late Mrs. Maxine E. Wright. It is also dedicated to the various health advocates of the past and present, people like the late Honorable Elijah Muhammad (the first renown propagator of nutrition), Dick Gregory, and many others. It is also dedicated to all those who are trying to change their diets and those who have achieved successful positive change. Congratulations.

Acknowledgments

I would also like to thank the following persons for their assistance Tim Morrow, Priscilla Flowers, Sandra Brooks, Eloise Prescott, Dr. Paul Bodhise, Dr. Fred Burton, Carol Mitchell, Tony Jackson, Swami Virato, Walter Morton and others whom I may have neglected to mention.

I hope that each and everyone who reads this humble contribution will be encouraged and enlightened and that they will then be motivated to put much of what is suggested into practical application.

Contents

From the Author

The purpose of this book is to enhance our knowledge of diet, food, and their related good habits so that we can improve our life. Additionally, we hope to offer valuable information on interrelationship between diet, mental health, the environment, and spiritual aspirations.

There is a great need for knowledge on health maintenance and nutrition. People desire more quality information about health topics. They wish to maintain their own health at an optimal level.

This book is written to inform everyone, from a meat eater and junk food person to a raw food vegetarian. It is a book that young, old, rich, poor, Christian, Muslim, Buddhist, or anyone can utilize and greatly benefit from now and in the future.

It is based on the good, better, and best principle. This principle says that you start out doing good, then you try to do even better so you can attempt to do the best. We all need to make transitions. This writing will tell us how.

The recipes contained in the last section of this book are delicious and easy to prepare. They represent the same high-nutritional standards that we provided to our customers at the Natural Oasis Restaurant in Philadelphia, Pennsylvania.

This book is written in a brief and concise manner for your convenience. The information it contains is the result of several hundred hours of research and reading. This involved attending seminars and conferences on wholistic health issues and meetings and discussions with a number of health related practitioners.

In the following pages we will explain the good, bad, and in-between of many foods. We hope to bridge the gap between meat-eaters and vegetarians. We will attempt to present the information in the most painless and palatable manner possible.

We want you to open up your minds and use your God given intuitive common sense as you read. That is your greatest tool in understanding and making transitions. It is our responsibility to take care of our bodies and we cannot delegate the responsibility to another (expert or not) without our own efforts.

We should know our bodies and how to maintain optimal health. When we have to go to our health professionals for aid or advice they may be the experts, but we should be knowledgeable participants in the process of attaining wellness. We can thereby reduce the possibilities of being misinformed or experiencing unnecessary pain, discomfort and/or cost.

Additionally, the scriptural quotes in this writing do not indicate a religious disposition. They only indicate that there is a respected (by many) reference point of the past that verifies and supports much of the information that is presented.

Introduction

Good health is important to all of us. There is much information on issues related to diet and health. Most of us want to know what is good for us and what is not. But we only want to alter what is necessary.

Wherever we are in terms of our diet we can always improve. To make transitions most of us read, talk to knowledgeable practitioners, and experiment with the various methods of attaining optimal wellness.

Most of us read several articles and books about dietary issues and health concerns before we add our own credence to information. Changing for the betterment of yourself is wonderful and exciting when you consider the positive consequences.

It can be challenging for some of us to change old habits and practices. But it is surely not difficult. There are many suggestions in this writing. And Confucius said, "every journey, no matter how long, starts with the first step."

I should know. Many years ago (20 years or more), in terms of diet I was probably in a similar situation with most people in America today. I ate pork and beef. I was a sugar junkie and labored over the main meal just to get to the cookies, cakes and pies. I consumed plenty of dairy products including milk, cheese, eggs, and margarine. I was slightly overweight and became a smoker.

When I went off to college, things started to change slowly. I matriculated at the University of Pennsylvania in the early 1970's. At that period in my life athletics and looking good were important. Although I wasn't an athlete, I wanted to look the part. After my hair began to gray and fall out, I became concerned.

I started making small changes in my diet because I wanted to be healthier. I stopped eating pork and didn't eat as much. I started eating more wholesome meals and I ate more fresh fruits. I started to exercise more. I noticed that I had more energy and felt better.

After graduating from college, I stopped eating all red meat. I began seriously to research nutrition and health issues. About 1981, I became a strict vegetarian and stopped eating dairy products, chicken, fish, or turkey except for two or three times a year. I began experimenting with non-meat recipes. I found that they tasted great and I didn't miss the meat.

Today as an iridologist, herbalist, and nutrition advocate, I am keenly aware of the relationship between food and health. When you mistreat your body temple with what you put into it, you will eventually pay a dear price. The same is true for the environment.

A brief word about Iridology, it is the science of evaluating the quality of health by looking in the iris of both eyes. It is a very valuable predictive tool that shows health problems and potential health problems. Each part of the eye corresponds to a different part of the body. By looking into the eye (with a glass loop and a light) and knowing the corresponding body parts, you can get more information about a person's health. Herbs and/or other treatments can then be suggested.

I believe that my experiences are valuable to those who want to learn what they can do independently to maintain and improve their health condition. Using Iridology, and the information I researched, I have been able to help many people who have had problems.

After some testing and experimenting, I have found the lifestyle which helps me to obtain optimal health. It is hoped that this writing will assist you in your search for the same. This writing can also help you avoid many of the pitfalls, clarify many of the contemporary health and dietary issues, and do so in a comprehensive and succinct manner.

This book is written to provide additional information on health and nutrition. It is not intended to replace your health professional (doctor, naturopath, chiropractor, or herbalist). I am not prescribing medicine or acting in the role of a doctor. If you follow the advice outlined in this book you are treating yourself, which is your right and privilege.

The Realities

"Behold I have given you every herb bearing seed which is upon the face of the earth and every tree in which is the fruit of a tree yielding seed; to you it shall be meat and to every beast of the earth, and to every fowl of the air and to everything that creepeth upon the earth, wherein there is life, I have given every green herb for meat, and it was so." Genesis 1:29-30.

Foods for Spirit

All life emanated spiritually from the breath of the Creator's presence. The breath is the manifestation of the inner force. The inner force is God's presence within our bodies. Almighty God nourishes us directly on the spiritual plane and indirectly on the physical and mental planes.

The mind is the great intercessor between the body and the spirit. Most people are not fully aware of the power of the mind over the body. The mind influences indirectly the state of health of the body. And thoughts create and form the mind. The great positive thinkers of yesterday and today all say that thoughts focused upon by the mind (good or bad) are what we become.

Our thoughts are greatly influenced by the foods we eat. Our diet affects every aspect of our life (physical, mental, and spiritual). It affects our emotions and even our sexual proclivities and abilities.

The body is a perfectly designed machine. It is so precise and exact that it could only have been Divinely created. Therefore doesn't your body deserve the best? Doesn't it deserve the best nourishment?

Food has great influence on our social and business life. Many business deals are consummated over food. Males and females get to know each other over food. Families and others relax and wind down over food. Important celebrations such as weddings, picnics, religious affairs, and fund raising efforts have food as the major facet of the event.

Even in scripture, food is a means of demonstrating fellowship and friendship. If we wish to show appreciation, affection, and hospitality, we should want to serve the best quality foods.

The advertising media, food retailers and producers have become our teachers on what foods are good or bad. The makers of foods that are high in sugar, saturated fats, cholesterol, and salt deceive us with deceptive and suggestively false advertising.

The fast food chains are the prime culprits, and huge profits are reaped at the public's expense. We suffer as our bodies begin to degenerate, our immune system breaks down, and our mental alertness wanes. We get fat and the aging process accelerates. Our energy level gets lower and lower.

Hippocrates, the father of Western medicine, said "let your food be your medicine and your medicine your food." We must gain nourishment from the same source as animals and plants, namely, Mother Nature (our mother) and the earth (our home). For we are a part of life's process, a continuum which guarantees us harmony, order, and perfection. If we do not adhere to certain rules, then we'll continue our downward spiral to self destruction.

Earthbound

The perfection and balance that exists on the earth plane is duplicated in the human body. The body has all 103 chemical elements that the earth possesses. The body needs fresh air, clean water, and life replenishing foods. The earth has all the necessary materials to sustain all of man's needs. But we must not continue to disrespect the earth and deplete her resources.

The natural state for the body is perfect health. The harmony and order of the body is supposed to be maintained by each individual. This can be successfully done by developing smart eating habits, taking food supplements, and exercising regularly. We can learn more by informative reading and discussions with knowledgeable people.

It is our natural right to live in an environment free of cancer-causing toxifying agents. Free of polluted air and of pesticide-laden foods. Free of hidden toxic waste dumps and polluted water. We only need to read the newspaper or watch the news to verify the pervasiveness of this reality.

Many of the so-called experts try to ignore the impact of these agents of ill health. But Mother Nature will not let us ignore it. There is a balance in the earth and in the body. Our mother constantly seeks this balance. The more imbalanced the earth (and the body) becomes through acts of men, the more Mother Nature seeks this balance. Even if nature must rearrange, knock over or destroy in the process, this balance will be achieved in time.

This is the first time in known world history that the environment has been so abused and plundered, yet so few people realize that the quality of life for all human beings is directly related to how we treat the environment. People have lost touch with nature and the natural balance outside of themselves. The ecological needs of the earth have been put below profit in grandiose fashion.

Why is it that we disrespect an earth that has been so good to us? Is greed, selfishness, and apathy that powerful in the environment? Do we understand that we will all pay for this disrespect of our home in one way or another?

In today's time payback is in process. Look at the depletion of the ozone layer. In most major metropolitan areas the air is really unfit to breathe. There are changes in climate and air quality mainly because of pollution and deforestation. A simple science lesson that we all should have learned is that plants and trees breathe in carbon compounds from automobiles, factories, etc. They then breathe out life giving oxygen. When you cut down trees you eliminate an important oxygen source and the means to decrease carbon compounds in the atmosphere.

Greedy farming corporations and smaller operators spray pesticides on our foods. Many foreign farming operators spray pesticides while the workers are in the fields. Food processors ignore the effects of overly processed foods. They put cancer-causing and health-debilitating preservatives in packaged, canned, and frozen products. This is the only society where people can make a joke about nuking their food in the microwave and the new threat is food irradiation.

Most of our cities water systems are unfit for human consumption (without a quality water filter). Corporations have dumped huge amounts of chemical poisons in our rivers and streams without concern for environmental impact.

The Bible says "What does it profit a man to gain the world and lose his soul?" Supplementing such a truism we say "Is it intelligent to produce wealth at the expense of your own ability to survive?" Money and wealth mean nothing if we are too sick or not even here to enjoy it. Do we think that all the diseases and health problems are just coming out of the sky? They are the result of our violating our bodies (with improper food and drugs) and disrespecting the earth.

There is a way back to the natural. It must be promulgated in the political, economic, and social realm. Our legislators must be fully cognizant of our desire to reverse the violations. We must make the growers, food processors, and food retailers more responsible through boycotts, exposure, and legal action.

We must encourage everyone and especially those in our households to become serious about health. Remember it's not just how long that you live, but also the quality of your health. We should be able to live in fairly good health until we are almost 100 years old, but only if we practice good eating habits and control our emotions.

If we are miserable then the God Force within us is likewise. And ability to fully express ourselves on this earth plane is abbreviated along with the human potential for the best. So when we eat, we are eating for today and tomorrow. We are nourishing our higher intelligence and our ability to energize ourselves.

Real Future Images

Can you envision the world as it once was and still can be, a reflection of the Garden of Eden? This would be a world where interdependence is acknowledged and nations, communities, families, and individuals respectfully and righteously exchange information for each other's mutual survival. A world where governments work together to cooperatively solve all the world's problems.

A world where America is striving to reach her potential and encouraging other nations to be self-sufficient and reach their potential. A world where the war machine psychology is mitigated by the many thoughts of the peace time challenges. A world where people de-emphasize the differences between each other and focus more on issues of common good.

Can you picture a land with pure unpolluted mountain streams, flowing into pure waters containing fish fit to be consumed if desired. A landscape designed with more green and trees to provide more oxygen and less carbon monoxide and dioxide.

There would be a health delivery system where the profit motive is de-emphasized and natures way is emphasized (herbs, food, vitamins, and homeopathic remedies). Can you imagine a political system that highly regards the environment and human health? A system that severely punishes any individual and/or corporation who disrespects, abuses, or deceives us about the environment.

Can you envision food grown without pesticides on soil, where the highest farming and ecological standards are observed? What about undepleted forests that are exploited only under the strictest ecological standards.

Can you envision a medical industry that emphasizes health prevention and wholisitic wellness instead of disease treatment and control of health conditions. An industry that uses modern technological advances and rational approaches to optimal health. An industry where greed and money needs are de-emphasized Can you imagine doctors being able to almost guarantee optimal health for the individuals that they treat?

With that kind of environmental concern we could make our food growing standards more reflective of the optimum health needs of all of us. All food would be grown organically. The food processors would again exact strict standards for their final food products. Hence they would eliminate all sugar and dangerous toxic drugs which preserve, color, or enhance foodstuffs.

The pesticide problem would disappear as innovations would help us to find new ways of protecting our crops without poisoning us. Alcohol, coffee, sugar, and tobacco consumption would be greatly decreased being replaced with herbal teas, natural juice beverages, and fresh air. Meats (beef and pork) would seldom be eaten and more emphasis would be placed on living goods such as: fruits, nuts, whole grains, vegetables, legumes, and herbs. People would eat more raw food and less cooked food.

The architects and engineers would develop a strong ecological perspective. They would work to improve the environment and their construction activities would reflect this. They would work with government not to construct buildings, roads, and parking lots on land that could be more efficiently used for food and agricultural products.

Nuclear weapons and power plants would be gradually done away with. As less meat is consumed, less energy is required. (A huge amount of our energy needs are devoted to growing and raising cattle and getting the final meat products to the marketplace.) Genetic engineers and food scientists would take a more wholistic and humane approach to food and drug experiments. They would revere and respect Mother Nature as the greatest chemist. They would be extremely cautious about tampering with natural processes.

Drug use (legal and illegal) would be drastically reduced as the social, economic, food, and spiritual problems become less. White refined sugar consumption would become extinct as people prefer more natural sweets. Stress and tension would be greatly reduced. Prisons and mental hospitals would operate at much less than capacity and many would close their doors.

A new attitude would have people replacing apathy, greed, jealousy, resentment, racism, and hatred with a new open spirit of positivism and intelligent vision. Differences would become less significant as cooperation takes its place. Crime would seldom occur because people would be more respectful of themselves, of others, and of their environment.

America would be more positive, more optimistic, and respected throughout the world as a true leader in promoting harmony. This spirit would inspire the world to bring about peace, sanity, justice, truth, intelligence, righteousness, and charity. Greed would be reduced to the lowest levels and giving becomes the trend.

Isn't this what we all want? Well, let us get busy and actualize this. It can be done. If we love humanity and want a better life for ourselves and our children we'll hurry to do it.

The Adversities

"He that overcometh (all desires of the flesh) shall inherit all things and I will be his guide and he shall follow me in health and happiness." Rev. 21:7.

Overviews

As was previously mentioned food plays a key role in our lifestyle. Many people eat three main meals a day. They have little concern for the quality of that food. They trust that the food is not harmful and if it is, "you've got to die from something," they say. Many of us live to eat. Eating is a favorite pastime.

Many of us are foodaholics with a legal addiction. We have pot bellies, don't exercise, eat bad food, wolf down wrong food combinations, and are over-stressed. We often feel weak, apathetic, and unalert. Our only prayer is to make it through another day, make some more money, and eat another meal.

Many people drown their frustrations with food. Some respond to their feelings of low self-esteem, dissatisfaction with themselves and their position in life and emotional reactions (anger, resentment, etc.) with what they put in their mouths.

Our mothers, although meaning well, introduced us to the foods that undo our healthiness later in life. Children are taught to eat what can be gobbled down quickly and what tastes good. Parents often times succumb to their children's insistence on eating good-tasting junk foods. Today's parents with so much to do tend to emphasize instantly prepared food. Most people eat microwave, chemicalized foods with little or no concern for their health until they get sick. And eventually they will get sick.

Sugar: How Sweet We Think it Is

Sugar is reported to be the number three killer in America (it's really the number two killer). It debilitates the body and the mind. White refined sugar that is. Sugar is actually another drug. It is turned white by a "bleaching" process, which involves using chemicals and, in some cases, pork by-products. If you desire good health and if you want control over yourself, don't use it. Overuse of sugar will eventually cause diabetic and pre-diabetic conditions (e.g., hypoglycemia).

Diabetes is a disease where the pancreas ceases to function properly. The job of the pancreas is to produce insulin that the body uses to transport glucose to the cells for energy. When too much sugar is consumed, the pancreas is overworked to produce enough insulin to metabolize the food consumed. The overworked pancreas creates a serious condition. If this serious condition persists, the result is hyperglycemia or diabetes. That's when the pancreas is producing much less insulin than necessary for your body to function properly. Eventually the pancreas will almost lose its ability to produce insulin. That's when artificial insulin is introduced.

Since the turn of the century, diabetes has increased tremendously (more than tenfold). Sugar is the main culprit. Sugar leeches calcium out of the body. Hypertension, heart problems, cancer, circulatory problems and several other health maladies can also be attributed to sugar. Its sweetness is deceptive but important. It can be related to a persons longing for the sweetness in life after enduring much conflict and dissatisfaction.

Sugar is an empty carbohydrate. It has no food value. It is not like the sugar cane (which it is derived from) which contains several vitamins and minerals. For in the process of producing sugar, it is stripped of nutrients. Sugar wreaks havoc on the heart, spleen, blood, brain, pancreas, adrenals, liver, and other organs. And a diabetic condition only means that the body can't take it anymore.

There are almost a half million insulin dependent diabetics in America. Insulin is a good example of how a typical drug or medicine affects the body. It supplies the body of a diabetic person with a life-saving substance necessary for energy and the proper digestion of our food. It is taken by injection in more severe (diabetic) cases.

However it is artificial (manmade) and cannot be as perfect as what the Creative Force makes. It does have potential side affects, namely, nausea, tiredness, and poor circulation. In other words insulin eventually can cause some of the problems it originally was intended to prevent. Insulin adversely affects sight, hearing, kidneys, memory, and teeth.

Sugar is put in most processed foods. Just go to the supermarket and read the ingredients in many food items. It is put in condiments (ketchup and relish), in most of the sodas and juices, and in commercial drink mixes (iced tea, punch, etc.). It is placed in just about all desserts (cookies, cakes, ice cream, etc.). It is the main ingredient in almost all candies and many breakfast cereals. It is in many food preparations, preservatives, and many foods that we are not aware of like pizza. It is in canned vegetable and fruit foods (fruit cocktail, sweet potatoes, etc.).

Corn syrup and high fructose syrup are two sweeteners that are processed and just as bad as sugar. Brown sugar is white refined sugar with molasses. Sugar is put in most cigarettes, some alcohol products, cough syrups, and many hospital drugs preparations. It is placed in many drugs (legal and illegal). Sugar is put in many illegal drugs. In fact sugar is more addictive than most of the drugs that contain it.

Sugar mollifies the immune system and tends to make us weak and lethargic. It disturbs the stomach and the digestive system. It robs the body of nutrients, most importantly the water soluble vitamins (B-complex and C). Vitamin C and the B-complex family are vital for managing stress, controlling the nerves, and the proper functioning of the brain.

It is no surprise to discover that the majority of people in mental institutions and jails are heavy sugar eaters. Also most people with general mind problems (e.g. depressive, schizophrenia, or paranoid) consume too much sugar. Most drug addicts and users have a sugar problem. Hyperactive and problem children can be brought back to normal by greatly reducing their sugar intake and giving them nervine herbs (e.g. hops, skullcap, valerian or catnip).

How could such a pernicious, health-deteriorating product be so accepted and widely used? First we must point to the advertising media and the food producers. Then we should look at the medical industry, which either ignores or greatly underestimates the power of this substance.

But another facet of its wide appeal and acceptance is its long history. Sugar has been around for at least 2000 years. It was once a delicacy desired by many of the powerful and affluent in certain parts of the world. It was at one time a very valuable and was a precious commodity. It became symbolic of wealth, affluence, and aristocracy. Wars have been fought over it.

Can you believe such a dangerous substance was so revered? Maybe then people didn't know, but today the information is available. One just has to look for it. There are several books written on the dangers of eating sugar. (See reference section at the end of this book.)

To reverse the effects of a sugar addiction or a diabetes condition, the first step is to clean the liver and the pancreas with a good herb (dandelion). Then you need a blood purifier (chaparral) and a colon cleanser (aloe, psyllium, senna, buckthorn or cascara sagrada), depending on the degree of constipation. Then you need a good vitamin and mineral supplement.

Beef and pork should be eliminated from the diet. Fish, turkey, and chicken can be consumed while changing the diet. But a vegetarian diet is better. Flesh free meals full of legumes, nuts, whole grains, fresh fruits, and vegetables will nutrify the body.

Caffeine should also be eliminated from the diet. The main products sold in America that contain caffeine (soda, coffee, and chocolate) also contain or are used with sugar. Caffeine, like sugar, robs the body of nutrients, disturbs digestion, and pollutes the blood, the kidneys, the heart, the liver, and the lymphatic system.

Caffeine is the number two addiction in America (of course sugar is number one). Caffeine is the largest cause of stomach cancer. And coffee is the main culprit of all the caffeine products. To break the caffeine habit, one must put nutrients back in the body. One should also take the herb dandelion to clean the liver and fortify the blood. Following the previously mentioned (pertaining to breaking the sugar habit) suggestions should be very helpful.

Stress, Sugar, and Mental Problems

Insanity and serious mental problems have increased fourfold in the past fifty years. More than ten percent of all Americans have some sort of serious mental problems. Many more have serious emotional problems that require counseling and/or drug treatment. Junk foods, primarily sugared foods, are the main culprits. Prolonged mind problems are accepted as normal. Stress and the related emotive reactions (anger, hurt, resentment) are examples.

Sugar leeches valuable nutrients out of the body. The B-complex family, vitamin C, and the minerals zinc and calcium are most important. Sugar disturbs the proper functioning of the liver and pancreas. It also interferes with metabolism, energy, motor ability, comprehension, and many of the brain functions.

Stress, depression, and anxiety are all precipitated by dietary toxins (bad foods), with sugar being a major culprit. All of these emotive reactions cause a further depletion of the B-vitamins which are vital to the proper functioning of the brain, spine, and the nerves. Vitamin C, the minerals zinc, calcium, and magnesium are also important during times of stress and sleeplessness. The herbs camomile, hops, valerian, and skullcap are excellent for managing stress, depression, anxiety, paranoia, and other mind problems.

Turbinado (natural) sugar and fructose (fruit sugar) are much better alternatives to white refined sugar but eating too much of them may produce some of the same problems. Pure honey is even better but over consumption of this good food can result in health problems. Pure, raw unfiltered honey is the better honey. Tupelo honey, maple syrup, carob, blackstrap molasses, and grain sweeteners are the best quality of sweets. Rice syrup and barley malt are examples of good grain sweeteners. Carob, a low calorie chocolate substitute has lots of calcium, potassium, phosphorus, vitamin A and some B vitamins.

Stress Defined

Stress can be defined as body or mental tension (pressure) induced by many factors such as lifestyle, environment, and occupation. Stress becomes a real potential health hazard when it is prolonged without a break for long periods of time. Although people handle prolonged stress differently, (some well, others not) it seems to have some adverse affects on us in the long term.

The great majority of Americans have too much stress in their lives. Bad reactions to stress can range from addictions (drugs, alcohol, tobacco, food) to negative physical responses such as abusing someone (wife, children), to health problems (ulcers, high blood pressure), and mental health problems (nervous breakdown, schizophrenia, insanity).

Our emotions are the reactants that determine how we handle stress. We all have emotions. But our ability to control our emotions will allow us to successfully overcome stressful situations. Eating the wrong foods with few nutrients will prevent us from being at our best in the battle to defeat stress. Eating good quality foods with sufficient nutrients and taking vitamins and herbs will equip us to do battle with stress. Almost every adverse health condition caused by stress is also caused by sugar (e.g. polluted blood, improper food digestion, increased heart rate and blood pressure, constipation, and mental abnormalities).

But foods are not the only problem. We must feel good about ourselves and have a good outlook on life. How we language (perceive and interpret) life determines our outlook.

Emotions and stress can be controlled. Think positive. Repeat positive affirmations (e.g. I will handle any problem that confronts me today). Meditation and prayer are important. Learn to think through situations. Laughter and being around positive (or friendly) people can help. Acknowledge the Creator's presence within you and dwell upon that.

Don't curse or you'll just make it worse. Cursing creates negative vibrations around you. Remember life is largely the picture that you create in your mind. Make your mind positive, productive, colorful, helpful, unselfish and true. Then the benefits will accrue.

The Heart

America has about seventy percent of the world's heart problems. Heart problems have increased thirty percent over the past fifty years. It has been reported that the American Heart Association estimates that there are about 1.5 million heart attack victims annually and over 500,000 of that number succumb. Heart disease cost over fifty billion dollars annually in health care and lost productivity costs. Heart disease is the nation's number one killer.

The heart is an amazing organ. It pumps or beats about 100,000 times every day. It pumps four quarts of blood throughout the body every minute. The heart pumps the blood through three types of vessels. These blood vessels are called arteries, veins and capillaries.

The arteries transport the blood which contains oxygen and nutrients (from our food) to the many cells in the body. Arteries break down into very small blood vessels called capillaries. The blood travels through the capillaries to the veins which then transport the blood back to the heart after the cells have been nourished. The veins also take away from the cells waste material (e.g. carbon dioxide).

The blood is composed of red and white cells. The red blood cells have as one of its components hemoglobin. Hemoglobin transports the oxygen to all parts of the body. Hemoglobin also gives blood its red color. White blood cells protect us from disease.

The heart and the blood directly affect each other. If the blood is polluted, it will weaken the heart and eventually put a great burden on it. Polluted blood is the cause of artery problems and it will adversely affect many of the body organs.

The heart, like other organs renews itself every year. Constantly the cells are created new. We get new blood every 90 days and new bones every 2 years. We get brand new cells for the heart, liver, kidneys, and other organs every 12 months.

Keep in mind the body is constantly rebuilding and renewing itself. Good foods facilitate in this process. Literally billions of cells die each day and others are created. When we eat right, all cells do their job as the Creator planned. Otherwise there are heartfelt problems.

The heart is the center of feeling. It is related to our emotions. That's why one aspect of avoiding heart problems is to avoid persistent tension and emotional imbalance. Stress is a contributor to heart problems. Arguing and conflict don't help the heart either.

To have a good heart one must avoid consumption of meat, most dairy products, white flour products, sugar, junk food, alcohol, drugs (legal and illegal), and cigarettes. Meats are the number one cause of a high cholesterol level, which is a precursor to heart problems. The cholesterol level is one way to gauge one's chances for a heart attack. We all have cholesterol in our bodies.

In a healthy body cholesterol is a clear mucous-like substance. When we eat bad foods, this substance thickens and changes color and becomes a residue of waste. In other words, cholesterol is a measurement of waste that cannot nutrify, enhance, or enliven the body. When we eat high cholesterol foods, (primarily animal products) we add waste to the body and the blood cholesterol rises.

The result is atherosclerosis which is the scarring, blockage, and weakening of the artery walls. Every other person that dies has a problem related to clogged arteries, and the great majority of Americans over fifty years of age (ninety percent) have arteriosclerosis which is essentially the same as atherosclerosis.

This problem not only causes heart attacks, but also strokes, senility, and poor circulation. It is the reason for bypass operations. But if you clean the plaque off the artery walls with good foods and herbs you can avoid bypass operations and heart trouble.

Animal flesh (especially beef and pork) cause special problems for the blood and the heart. Too much animal protein increases the acid in the body and thickens the blood, putting a strain on the arteries and the heart. Contrary to generally accepted beliefs, meat is not essential for health and strength. In fact, meat decreases endurance, strength, and your quality of health.

Animal flesh, especially beef and pork, have uric acid in them. Uric acid is urine from the animal. It is the waste from living tissues. Normally this waste is delivered by the blood to the kidneys. It would then be passed on to the bladder and then eliminated.

When the animal is killed the uric acid is still in the flesh. It makes the meat toxic. It pollutes the blood and the heart. It causes arthritis, gout, kidney troubles, and other health problems. But ironically the uric acid (urine) gives some flavor to the meat.

The other health problem with all flesh (beef, pork, fish, fowl, etc.) is the harmful bacteria that it contains. The putrefactive bacteria or germs enter the body of the animal from the colon after it is killed. These germs if consumed will pollute the blood and hence affect the heart especially in the case of pork and beef.

But this bacteria has been found in large concentration in all animal flesh. And cooking the flesh may not destroy the germs. However, if you stop eating flesh or greatly reduce your consumption and take certain herbs (e.g. chaparral, cayenne, red clover, or fresh garlic) the blood can be cleansed and the heart strengthened in a short period of time. Remember non-meat eaters (vegetarians) tend to be healthier than meat eaters.

The body can heal itself. Almost every disease and health problem can be treated. And high cholesterol and heart problems are no different. The low cholesterol or cholesterol free foods are whole grains, fresh vegetables, legumes, and fruits. These foods will actually lower the cholesterol level.

Salt deserves special mention as a contributor to heart problems. It pollutes the blood stream and irritates the stomach. Salt cannot be effectively digested and used by the body. Salt is addictive and health damaging. It can also cause cancer. It disguises the taste of foods and trains the taste buds to be anticipating its taste. Most fast food restaurants oversalt the foods and meats are cured with salt. Salt consists of sodium and chloride but these minerals are not in a form readily usable by the body. There is a good amount of sodium in most vegetables and fruits which is usable and good for the body. Sea salt is a better alternative to regular salt.

The majority of animal products (e.g. beef, pork, dairy products, chicken) and white flour products are high in cholesterol and saturated fats. Saturated fats also cause heart attacks. Very few vegetable fats are saturated. Coconut oil, palm oil, and hardened oil are the only exceptions.

Safflower oil is one of the great oils which is unsaturated. Olive oil, sunflower oil, sesame oil, and corn oil are also unsaturated. Research has been completed on the benefits of fish oils and olive oil in lowering cholesterol levels. Oats, oatmeal, and oat bran have been found to reduce cholesterol levels and heart problems. Lecithin aids in reducing the cholesterol level.

The circulatory system (blood) must be kept clean and flowing to avoid heart problems. Eat plenty of raw fruits and vegetables. Take herbs such as fresh garlic and cayenne pepper.

Exercise done properly will help strengthen the heart muscle. Walking is a great exercise that most of us can do. Jogging, bicycling, and swimming are also good. Aerobics and general calisthenics are great too.

Check with your health advisor (doctor, chiropractor, nutritionist, etc.) to be assured of the safety of the exercise program.

The Digestive System

The digestive system may be the most important body system. It is amazing and wonderful. It starts at the mouth and ends at the rectum. In between there are many organs that are vital to processing the foods that we eat. These organs also provide nourishment for the cells, and facilitate the elimination of the waste.

The mouth and chewing starts the process. There are certain enzymes that are secreted in the mouth which help digestion. We have to chew our food enough times (e.g. 30 times a bite) for the enzymes to effectively start the process of breaking our food down. Then the food enters the stomach which is the physical intelligence center. The stomach starts the food absorption and breakdown process. The stomach has hydrochloric acid which actually breaks down the food.

The stomach breaks down the food and then decides how to distribute it throughout the body. It sends the nourishment to the proper areas and places the remainder of the unused food into the intestines. The small intestine takes the life out of the food and puts it into the bloodstream to give us energy and nutrients. It's about 25 feet long. Then the remainder of the food is pushed along through the large intestine and into the colon. At this point it is mainly waste.

The food enters the colon through the ileocecal valve. The remaining minerals are absorbed in the colon and the waste pushed along up the ascending colon across the transverse colon down the descending colon, and out the rectum.

Stress and bad foods (caffeine, sugar, junk foods, etc.) disturb the stomach. When the improper foods are consumed, the stomach cannot do it's job effectively and the cells do not get proper nourishment. The waste moves along very slow, resulting in constipation. The circulatory system becomes polluted because the waste build-up begins to leak into it. This process toxifies and overtaxes the body organs and systems. The result is disease.

Even a cold and a flu are the body's reacting to the toxins within it. In a sense, a cold is a blessing for it gives the body the opportunity to get this waste out of it. In fact, the best remedy for the common cold (or flu) is to clean the system, clean the colon, and give the body it's vital nutrients.

Golden seal, peppermint, or mullein clean the system. Cascara sagrada, aloe vera, or senna clean the colon. Carrot juice, rose hips (natural vitamin C), and a good diet (and food additives) will nutrify the body. Peppermint tea with lemon and pure, unfiltered honey is a good remedy for colds and flu. It can be taken along with the above mentioned foods and herbs. Adding garlic (chewing or in food) or cayenne pepper (in food) enhances one's ability to get well soon. Additionally, gargling with cayenne pepper and/or lemons diluted in water are good remedies for a sore throat.

As you can see, the digestive system affects the entire body. When the blood no longer can nourish the system, either because of poor quality foods or stomach imbalance, the organs get weaker. They become vulnerable to health maladies. And dirty blood puts a greater strain on all body systems since the blood carries the waste and drops it off along the way in a polluted body.

One of the primary places that waste is deposited is in the lymphatic system. Throughout your body there are lymph nodes. They absorb a great deal of the waste in the body, but they too have a breaking point.

Americans spend several billion dollars a year on medication (e.g. antacids) to alleviate digestive disorders. Digestive disorders and constipation affect the blood, the adrenal glands, the lymphatic system, the endocrine system and the respiratory system. They both influence our sleeping patterns, energy level, sexual desires, temperament and our emotions. They both will cumulatively affect the skin and the liver.

The liver is the largest gland in the body and the largest organ in mass size. It weighs between forty and sixty ounces depending on the person. It is an important organ for many body processes including digestion. The liver filters much of the waste, but when it is overburdened, it loses its vitality. The liver is one of the most powerful regenerative organs of the body. It breaks down and absorbs many of our body wastes. It is a major organ of metabolism. It regulates carbohydrate, fat, and protein processing and stores vitamins and minerals.

The liver is also a regulator of blood sugar, producing glucose and glycogen. When you pollute your system with bad food, alcohol, drugs, and cigarettes, you impair this organ's ability to defend you. It takes a very long time for this organ to finally give out. And it is difficult to reverse a chronic liver problem. But by changing your diet and taking liver cleansing herbs (dandelion or barberry), the liver can be revived.

Enemas and colonic irrigations are an effective means of cleansing the colon and enhancing colon health. It involves putting pure water (and possibly herbs) into the colon through the rectum. The water is allowed to circulate through the colon and loosen the impacted waste in the colon. The waste and the water is then eliminated.

A colonic is very similar to an enema. In fact it is called a high enema. A colonic, generally speaking, follows the same colon cleansing process as an enema. And an enema can be done in the privacy of your home (with an enema tube and bottle). The enema only cleanses the rectum and descending colon area. These are the first areas to hold the waste buildup in the body.

An enema or colonic are useful tools in colon health, but herbs and proper foods are the foundation. Herbs will clean out the entire body including the colon and herbs will enhance the digestive process. The colon will cleanse itself (eventually) with an optimal diet consisting of lots of fruits and raw salads. Vegetables and whole grains are also important.

A person who is in the process of changing their diet (after years of eating improper foods) may want to get one or two colonics. But they should do so only after taking colon cleansing herbs for thirty to sixty days. A colonic takes the good and bad bacteria out of the colon. The good bacteria is necessary for proper elimination. It must be replaced or constipation may ensue.

Acidophilus is an excellent herb for replacing the good bacteria. It also enhances elimination and aids digestion.

High fiber foods are an important ingredient in a healthy lifestyle. High fiber foods enhance our digestive system and colon since they easily and quickly pass through our bodies. High fiber foods are unprocessed, unrefined, whole foods in their natural state. Most fruits, legumes and vegetables and all whole grains have high fiber.

Although the entire food contains fiber, the majority of the fiber is located in the outer covering of the grain or fruit or legume. This is where the greatest amount of nutrition is located. When the grain is refined the fiber is removed.

Most Americans east much less fiber than they should. In fact, the average Western diet consists of too much refined foods. This causes constipation, hemorrhoids and several other health problems. High fiber foods helps accelerate the process of digestion. They also can hold a good amount of water, making it easier to eliminate the waste of the colon. High fiber foods help the heart, the blood, the lymphatic system, the digestive system and many other body organs.

Additionally, high fiber foods aid in the cure of diabetes, cancer, obesity and many other health problems.

Other Eliminative Organs

Besides the colon there are three other important eliminative organs. They are the skin, the lungs and the kidneys.

The skin is the protective layer of the body. It protects the body from invading bacteria. The skin is so important that without it we could die quickly. It is the largest eliminative organ of the body. It is a powerful sensor, since it senses (detects) touch, pain, cold, and heat.

It is made up of two layers which are the outer layer, which is the epidermis and the dermis, which is the lower layer. Hair follicles grow out of the dermis through the epidermis.

The visible skin is made up of dead cells. New cells are continuously being created. The new cells are continuously rising to the outer layer and the dead cells slowly drop off the surface of the skin.

The color of the skin varies because of the melanin that is produced by the epidermis. The melanin can protect you from overexposure to the sun's rays. It also maximizes the amount of the sun's energy that our bodies can receive. The sun not only gives our bodies physical nourishment but also provides our minds with higher energy.

The skin is a temperature regulator for the body. The skin also allows you to sweat. Sweating allows your body to rid itself of toxins. Additionally, the skin manufactures some vitamin D from sunlight.

There are several kinds of skin problems. The main problems with skin are bumps and blemishes. Many people have acne, psoriasis, boils, bumps, eczema, itching, discolorations, warts, and blackheads. Essentially, these problems are caused by the inability of the body to eliminate toxins.

Putting it another way, when you eat too many bad foods, your body will try to eliminate a large percentage of the residual waste. If it can't efficiently do this (because the body processes are adversely affected when we don't eat enough good foods) then the waste will tend to collect around the areas where it usually eliminates. Since the skin is the largest organ of elimination, it may be directly and adversely affected.

Two other serious problems usually associated with bad skin are a toxic liver and polluted blood. The liver is one of the organs that filters the waste in the body. The blood carries the nutrients to the body areas and carries the waste away.

When we eat too many bad foods, our blood is overloaded with waste and our liver becomes toxic. A skin problem may be just a warning, for the problem might be putting us in an ominous plight.

To eliminate skin problems, one has to work on the actual visible problem and also the internal problem. There are salves, herbs, and ointments for the outside. There are herbs and foods which can have a positive affect on skin problems.

Aloe vera, olive oil, cocoa butter, lemons, lavender and anything with vitamin E (e.g. avocados), can be used externally. Aloe vera, red clover, yellow dock, chickweed, dandelion, redmond clay, and rose hips can be used internally.

Changing the diet is important too. One must greatly reduce the consumption of junk foods (mainly sugared junk foods). Eating less meat, less dairy products, and less processed foods are very important.

Skin problems are sometimes difficult to resolve. Just be patient and keep trying the herbs. These problems take diligent efforts to solve, but they do work. And don't forget to change your diet. Read the herb reference section for the herbs that may work for you.

The lungs receive air through the nose and the mouth. The air goes through the trachea (windpipe) to the bronchi. The bronchi feed into the lungs through small bronchioles which lead to a group of tiny air sacs called alveoli. The alveoli allow the oxygen to enter each cell in the lungs and the blood. The oxygen combines with glucose (a by-product of our foods) to produce energy. The energy is released. This is called respiration.

There are literally millions and millions of alveoli. They not only bring the oxygen to the blood but they also take away the blood carbon dioxide, water, and other waste products to be eliminated by the lungs.

The diaphragm encases the lungs for protection. It actually moves when you breathe. In other words when you breath, it actually contracts and expands. It is composed of a group of muscles vital to several body processes, the most important of which is breathing.

The lungs are depleted essentially by mucous (caused by bad foods). Mucous (waste) is primarily produced by dairy and white flour products, sugar, meat and processed foods. When you eat these foods the waste that these foods create cannot be eliminated by other means. So the lungs become a possible depository for this waste.

One can eliminate this waste by proper breathing, exercising, colon-cleansing, and lung-healing herbs. When all the eliminative organs are working properly then none of them can become overtaxed.

A brief word about smoking. Smoking (cigarettes, cigars, marijuana, etc.) is devastating to the lungs. The American Cancer Society estimates that there will be 178,100 new cases of lung cancer in 1997.

Smoking minimizes the amount of oxygen that the body can get by breathing. It also interferes with the expelling (when you exhale) of all the waste products that the lungs must rid the body of (e.g. carbon dioxide, water, and so forth). Smoking contributes to the mucous deposits in the lungs and helps diminish their vitality. It interferes with breathing and scars and discolors the lungs. Combine smoking with a bad diet and you will soon have serious trouble. So get rid of the smoking habit. The herbs catnip, skullcap and peppermint are very good herbs for one who desires to stop smoking.

Congested lungs (mucous), pneumonia, emphysema, and lung cancer are examples of lung maladies. Comfrey, eucalyptus, mullen, lobelia, slippery elm, and many other herbs help lung problems.

Breathing polluted air and smoking pollute the lungs. Lung cancer (mainly caused by smoking) is the number one cancer-causer. Lung congestion, coughs and colds are other problems. All can probably be eliminated by following the advice contained within, controlling habits, and using our God-given common sense.

The kidneys are another important eliminative organ. They get rid of the liquid waste, primarily water. They also get rid of other wastes. The kidneys also help balance out the level of water and salts in the body, and rid the body of carbon dioxide, a by-product of respiration.

Normally everyone has two kidneys. There is one on the left side and one on the right side. They are located in the lower back area.

The kidneys are a powerful filtering agent like the other eliminative organs. By controlling the body water level, the kidneys have a direct influence on weight.

When you drink water, your kidneys produce urine. The more or less water that we drink the more or less that we urinate. If you eat wrong foods and a lot of spices, drink too much coffee, soda and especially alcohol, the kidneys are affected adversely. They can become polluted and overtaxed. The subsequent problems could manifest themselves as infections, kidney stones, cancer, or the kidneys may even stop functioning. In the latter case a kidney machine might be used. But nature provides answers to just about all health maladies.

The herbs cornsilk, dandelion, juniper berries, marshmallow, and uva ursi help most kidney problems. Foods like lemon, watermelon, and cranberries are excellent for the kidneys.

The Colon, Overeating, and Overweight

The colon is a significant determinant of body health. It is one of the areas where there are nerve endings. Nerve endings are areas where you can determine the quality of health. The eyes, the hands, and the feet also contain nerve endings.

The colon's normal shape is an inverted U. 29

(See Illustration on page 123.) When we eat improperly, the colon loses its shape. This indicates that the colon is unhealthy and has lost its vitality. The person, by that time is suffering from severe constipation. Constipation is the failure to establish regular bowel movements. It is directly related to the improper functioning of the digestive system. It is also related to a decrease in the peristalsis action of the colon.

Peristalsis is the wavelike alternating contractions and dilations that move the waste through the colon. Peristalsis may not occur because improper eating taxes the digestive system and results in constipation. Consequently bowel movements are very sluggish. Since we eat the same amount but eliminate less frequently, the waste backs up in the body. The bloated waste-filled body eventually results in one of the many health problems. The blood becomes polluted.

Usually sickness or ill-health attacks our body at the weakest point. Improper elimination and bad foods debilitate the entire body. And the polluted blood loses it's ability to carry the nutrients to the entire body as well as the ability to take the waste from the body to it's elimination points. The body becomes weaker and weaker. Parasites wreak havoc in various parts of the body. Colorectal, cancer, hemorrhoids, and related disorders affect millions of Americans. Colorectal cancer is the second most prevalent cancer.

Americans spend over 300 million dollars annually on laxatives. Commercial laxatives are a very poor way to move the bowels. Laxatives create convulsions in the colon which moves the bowels along by causing expansions and contractions. This is not a natural pushing of the waste along through the colon, which is what the herbs do. Also, when the unnatural laxatives are discontinued the same constipation problem will recur (more than likely) and probably be worse. Optimally we should have a bowel movement within two to six hours after we eat. If it takes eight to eighteen hours, that may be satisfactory. But if it takes longer you may need some herbal assistance. Take a closer look at the diet to determine how to speed up elimination. The better the elimination is, the better potential the body has for optimal health.

Several herbs help digestion and elimination. Papaya, fennel, and acidophilus are digestive aids. Herbs for proper elimination and constipation include: aloe vera, buckthorn, acidophilus, senna, psyllium, and cascara sagrada.

A cleansing fast can help to insure good elimination. Prune juice, lemons, and carrot juice are fine. A one-day-a-week fast with quality juices, lemons, and maybe even enemas is great for the digestive system. Exercise is very important to achieve and maintain proper elimination. A simple walk of a few blocks thirty minutes after eating is fine.

The foods to avoid for good elimination are meats, fried foods, overly processed foods, dairy products, white sugar and white flour products. White flour products form a paste-like substance on the walls of the colon and intestines. This makes constipation an ongoing reality. Foods that enhance elimination are fresh vegetables (raw if possible) and fresh fruits. The specific foods that are good for proper elimination are apples, bran, figs, ginger, prunes, seeds, and grains especially millet and oatmeal.

So far we have discussed the digestive system and the colon. One may say, what does that have to do with obesity? Everything and more. When the digestive system is not functioning properly, waste accumulates in the body. We don't efficiently use or eliminate what we eat. For example, we may eat daily three pounds of food; the body may use efficiently one pound, we may eliminate one and a half pounds and one-half pound lingers in the body as unusable matter (waste).

The waste fills up the colon. The bowels move slower and slower. This waste pollutes the blood. The blood carries the waste to various parts of the body and drops it off. The favorite places to drop the waste are the buttocks, hips, thighs, stomach, and chest (or breast).

The bloated stomach is largely due to the colon filling up and losing its shape. Its normal shape becomes perverted. All sorts of illnesses set in. Most overweight people have a thyroid problem. This can be partially attributed to waste accumulation which is related to eating the wrong foods and overeating. The thyroid controls the rate of metabolism. This is directly related to the rate and amount of the food that we eat that is used to nutrify the body. Some foods slow metabolism (poor quality foods) while others increase it (good quality foods).

Over 75 million Americans are overweight. Over 36 million of that number are excessively obese. A huge number of heart attack and stroke victims as well as diabetics are overweight. Hypertension, lack of energy, and cancer (especially colon cancer) are associated with obesity. Obesity is also socially unappealing and can have negative psychological reactions (low self esteem).

It is not easy to lose weight, but it is not difficult either. Motivating a person to change bad habits is key. And cleansing the colon is first and foremost. We must eat whole foods (high fiber) to enhance proper bowel action. If elimination improves, all body organs tend to work better. The blood will tend to cleanse itself and the person looks and feels healthier. Drinking good amounts of water (e.g. 10-12 glasses daily) is very important in any weight loss program.

Exercise most definitely helps elimination. The first thing it does is get the blood circulating. This tends to activate the other eliminative organs such as the kidneys, the lungs, and the skin (the largest eliminative organ). When we sweat, we are eliminating toxins (waste). Our body thanks us by making us feel better.

When laxatives and some of the eliminative herbs are taken for long periods of time (e.g. three years) the bowels may tend to become a little sluggish if one stops taking them. The probable cause is that much of the good bacteria have been removed with the bad bacteria from the walls of the colon. The good bacteria are necessary for proper elimination. Acidophilus and quality foods (raw fruits, fresh vegetables and high fiber grains) put the good bacteria back in the colon and restore proper elimination.

Acidophilus may also be used after enemas or colonic irrigations. Acidophilus helps enhance the nutrient absorption and the intestinal flora (flora is the good bacteria). This helps move the waste along quickly and more efficiently. Hence the body becomes detoxified.

Acidophilus helps with digestive problems (e.g. indigestion and stomach problems). Acidophilus also helps lower the cholesterol level and eliminates bad breath. It comes in herb form and is also in yogurt. However most commercial yogurt is made with sugar and dairy products.

Underweight and Health

Most of us would agree that thinner people look better than overweight people. But are thin people healthier?

There may be a tendency to argue in the affirmative since overweight people are placing an excessive burden on the heart and other organs. However the health status of thin people can also be poor.

Have you ever heard a thin person say something like "I eat like a horse and can't seem to gain weight." Have you ever wondered why?

Many thin people have a high rate of metabolism. This means in brief that the food that they consume is more efficiently processed by the body. But if they eat bad foods, they can still be constipated and have the problems associated with constipation. And the liver and digestive system can be polluted, possibly causing an appetite reduction. Also stress and drugs can create an imbalance in the entire system (especially the liver) which can result in an appetite reduction.

Another important reason why people may be excessively thin is because they have parasites helping them to consume their food. Parasites are live organisms that enter the body through our regular eating. They can come from eating fruits and vegetables, but that is unusual. The main way that most of us get them into our bodies is by consuming animal products, primarily beef and pork.

Parasites also can be consumed through eating chicken and fish. They thrive and survive on animal products, white sugar, white flour products and all other bad foods. These bad foods turn into waste in the body and the parasites consume this waste.

To substantiate what I am saying, it is a well known fact that the trichinosis worm in pork can survive cooking and can be ingested alive. Also many of us who have had (or have) cats or dogs know that they can have worm problems. Well if they can get worms, what about humans?

Additionally, an iridologist can most likely observe the effects of parasites by looking in the eye (with a glass loupe). Also more and more health professionals, (including doctors) are very aware that parasites exist in the body and can cause all sorts of problems.

Parasites can wreak havoc in the body and damage certain organs causing a variety of health problems. Some of these problems are: heart and lung troubles, kidney, bladder, genital, digestive problems, colds, cancer, vision and brain abnormalities.

Parasites can exist in children, adults and senior citizens. Although excessively thin people are more obvious victims of parasites, they can be present in anyone. Their cumulative adverse affects usually become apparent in the middle years. More adolescents and younger adults are experiencing health problems that are directly or indirectly related to the damage that parasites have done.

By no means are we saying that all excessively thin people have parasites. However, if you eat bad foods or have only been eating properly for a short period of time, chances are you have parasites.

Parasites can live in the body for long periods of time, grow and multiply. They survive primarily off the bad foods that we eat. In other words, if you eat high quality foods, the parasites have difficulty surviving. And if one takes parasite-killing herbs, these worms will be destroyed and eliminated out of the body. The following herbs are very good for eliminating parasites, namely, black walnut, fresh garlic, pumpkin seeds, sage, wormwood and others.

There are several herbs which help one to gain weight. Camomile, ginseng, golden seal, strawberry and alfalfa will increase the appetite.

The Lymphatic System

The lymphatic system is a very important system in body functioning. The lymphatic system contains lymph nodes. The lymph nodes are primarily located where the body can bend, turn, or joins with another part. Some of the lymph nodes are in the neck, arms, chest, legs, inner thighs, and stomach. We normally have up to forty-five pints of lymphatic fluid in our bodies.

The lymphatic system is actually the immune system. This system protects us from toxins that come in the body. The lymphatic system helps to maintain the correct fluid balance in the tissues and blood, to conserve protein, and to remove bacteria and other cellular waste products. The lymphatics are made up of tiny vessels which circulate a milky fluid throughout the body. This is a very intricate filtering system that always defends us from toxins.

The lymphatic system and the circulatory system are closely interrelated. In fact, the two systems connect through valve openings in the thoracic duct. This duct extends from the abdomen area to the neck. It allows the lymphatic system to pick up and deliver materials (nutrients and waste) from the circulatory system.

Certain white blood cells are stored in the lymphatic system, namely, lymphocytes and phagocytes. When we get ill both are released into the blood stream to fight the illness. They will go anywhere in the body to fight the illness. The lymphocytes' job is to contain the spread of the disease (bacteria) so that the phagocytes can render them harmless by consuming them.

The lymphatic system also catches most of the excess mucous (waste) from our bad diet. The waste is delivered by the blood stream to the various lymph nodes. The lymph nodes store the waste. Then they release the waste into the bloodstream to be eliminated out the body. When we have a diet consisting mostly of bad foods, the lymphatics tend to collect more and more of the waste. The blood becomes polluted and loses its ability to eliminate the toxins. As we get older we cumulatively impair the lymphatics ability to fight the toxins.

Hence disease or illness sets in. Cancer and AIDS are two well-known diseases that are the result of a weakened immune system. They are actually the body's ultimate reaction to our violations of it. But we get warnings along the way. A cold, sinus problem, skin problem, constipation are all advanced warnings. And we usually try to ignore them until it's too late.

The Brain, The Spine, The Nervous System and Stress

The brain, the spine and the nervous system are interconnected and interdependent. What happens to one can directly affect the other. They are composed of a group of organs and/or tissues which transmit energy throughout the body and perform various bodily functions.

We will briefly and simply describe the important organs and systems. Primarily we want to show how stress and improper eating affects them.

The brain is the control center for the body. It is the source of energy for the body both electrical (or electronic) and spiritual. Electronic impulses are transmitted throughout the body from the brain through the nervous system. This allows the body to perform most activities both voluntary (talking, walking) and involuntary (breathing and heartbeat).

The spiritual energy is your higher consciousness energy or the cosmic (universal) energy that guides, directs and motivates the body. This energy also helps you to make choices and decisions. Our intunement with our spirit selves is a significant ingredient in our higher mental evolution, in controlling emotions, and in acquiring knowledge.

The brain consists of the following parts. The cortex is the large covering for the brain, which directs voluntary actions. The medulla (lower middle) controls involuntary actions. The cerebellum (below cortex) is a message transmitter and receiver for your muscles and various organs. The hypothalamus and thalamus (middle of brain) are distributors of energy throughout the body.

The brain needs physical nourishment. It requires certain nutrients from the foods that we eat and oxygen for the life of the cells. Without both of these brain cells may die. And the brain may atrophy, directly affecting our body's functioning and our ability to think and handle stress.

The B-complex vitamins are especially important for the brain. And all the other nutrients (vitamins, minerals and amino acids) are important too.

The herbs gota kola, eyebright, parsley, rose hips and alfalfa enhance the brain and have high amounts of the B-complex vitamins. The herbs alfalfa, chlorophyll, black walnut, blessed thistle and hawthorn have high amounts of oxygen and the B-complex vitamins. Oxygen is extremely vital to the functioning of the brain. Since the blood carries the oxygen, it is important that the head area have good blood circulation.

The brain is directly connected to the spinal cord through the brain stem. The spine is in the center of the back. It extends from the skull, down the vertebrae in the back, (which protects the spine) and ends at the coccyx (right above the buttocks).

The great majority of back and spine problems can be successfully treated with herbs and/or chiropractic treatments. Even ruptured discs can be treated without the necessity of surgery. The herbs valerian, wood betony, comfrey, alfalfa, and cayenne aid in problems with the back. Cayenne is good for so many problems because it enhances circulation and strengthens the blood.

Herbs with plentiful calcium and some vitamin C such as dandelion, rose hips, plantain, kelp, and yellow dock will help back problems. These herbs will aid in healing strains, sprains, muscle pulls, and fractures in most places in the body. Also posture is very important in maintaining a healthy back spine and nervous system. Stand and sit erect to avoid problems.

The spine and back can be injured fairly easily if one is under stress. Stress keeps the muscles tight and makes them susceptible to injury. A simple fall or slip, a wrong twist, turn, or strain while exercising, or a bad sleeping position can cause a few weeks or months of discomfort in the back. An over-stressed body possibly has several blockages where the energy flow has been obstructed. This too can cause pain. Herbs with chiropractic adjustments can resolve this problem.

The brain, the spine and the nerves form a complex message network in the body. They transmit, receive and relay various messages or signals. Some of the messages that they transmit include movement, pain, hunger, and touch.

The nervous system can be divided into the central nervous system and the peripheral nervous system. The central nervous system works through the spinal cord and the brain to monitor and regulate the majority of our body functions.

The peripheral nervous system connects organs and tissues not directly affected by the central nervous system to the central nervous system. The autonomic nervous system is a part of the peripheral nervous system. It controls the automatic body functions that are involuntary such as breathing, heartbeat, and digestion.

When one eats properly, takes extra nutrients, exercises, doesn't expose the body or the mind to traumas and controls their stress level, the nervous system (and its constituent parts) would be functioning at an optimum. If not, things can become very nerve-wracking.

All of the aforementioned foods that pollute the body (animal products, white flour products, refined sugar) and all drugs eventually will damage the brain and the nervous system. Significant imbalances in energy flow and message relay can occur. This can not only alter the nerve function, but also the areas of the body that the nerves are connected to, such as the back or shoulder. In fact, many spine and back problems are related to stress and an imbalanced nervous system.

Structural and bone problems can cause problems in the nervous system and visa versa. For example one may exercise and may have a back or ankle sprain because of improper eating and a stress-filled life. And improper eating is the main promoter of stress.

Remember when you eat improperly your brain cannot get the proper nutrients and its ability to receive life-giving oxygen is minimized. This can lead to many health problems. The number one problem it can immediately cause is stress. And stress can lead to heart, lung, kidney, skin and bowel problems. Stress is also the cause of many mental problems and mind abnormalities.

In America stress and unresolved emotional conflicts are very prevalent. Most people who work have job-related stress and tension. Trying to satisfy your supervisor or a customer, meeting deadlines, job security, not getting your proper rest, a possible promotion and wage problems are possible reasons for this stress.

Emotional conflicts are significant contributors to stress and tension. Emotional problems may initially occur during infancy and sometimes even in the mother's womb. There may be resentment, hatred, a traumatic experience or ill feelings (possibly towards the husband or mate) brewing inside the mother that could directly affect a baby or unborn child. And that child could carry that conflict (and others) for a lifetime.

Other people with conflicts may have had something traumatic happen to trigger their emotional troubles. Bad experiences such as molestation, violence, constant arguing, conflict and cursing in the home and/or witnessing a terrifying act can create emotional imbalance and negativity.

If a person acknowledges their problem, there are several methods of identifying and resolving an individual's latent emotional conflicts. But many times cumulative emotional conflicts trigger a violent and/or extremely anti-social reaction. Drug addictions are one possible result of this reality.

The prisons, drug rehabilitation centers, and mental hospitals are full of individuals with chronic stress and mind problems. The experts (psychiatrists, psychologists, counselors, and therapists) feel that serious mental problems can only be controlled with drugs and counseling. Although in some instances this may be true, the majority of mental maladies can be successfully treated without drugs. Proper diet is the foundation. Building an individual's level of self-esteem and enhancing a sense of purpose in life are important too. Learning how to express and language (interpret) conflict are important too.

The diet for people with these problems has been mentioned several times in this writing. First, eliminate white refined sugar. Most people with mental, drug or criminal problems have a sugar addiction. Sugar weakens the body and the mind and is the main stress producing food.

Reduce you consumption of flesh (especially beef and pork), dairy products, and white flour products. Eliminate tobacco, alcohol and other drugs (legal and illegal). If one is taking medication to control the problem, very gradually replace the drugs with herbs and do so with the advice of a knowledgeable health professional (e.g. herbalist, nutritionist, chiropractor, or doctor).

Eat quality foods such as fresh fruits, vegetables, legumes, and whole grains. Take extra nutrition supplements, especially the B-complex vitamins and vitamin C. Besides the herbs already mentioned, there are many herbs for the nerves. Hops, valerian, skullcap, catnip, lobelia and camomile are excellent for the nerves. If you can calm the nerves and eat properly, the brain can rejuvenate itself. And the muscles, the back and the spine are then less susceptible to sprains, strains, pulls and other more serious problems.

Cancer

Cancer is the body's reaction to physical and mental imbalance. Physically, it is over-production of abnormal cells due to improper diet. It is also the inability of the cells to regenerate themselves due to the accumulation of mucous (the by-product of processed foods). It usually affects the body's weakest organs. Mentally, it is related to unresolved stress and feelings of resentment. Cancer was rarely heard of years ago but today it is increasing at an alarming rate. It is estimated that twenty-five percent of the American public will get cancer in some form.

A general state of toxicity pervades the body when cancer exists. This toxicity is caused by consumption of improper foods such as: white sugar, coffee, tea, cola drinks, dairy products, meat (primarily pork and beef), white flour products, processed foods, overeating fried and heavily salted foods, and denatured foods. Also tobacco, alcohol, drugs (legal and illegal), polluted air and water, can lead to various forms of cancer.

Cancer can occur almost anywhere in the body, but the most likely areas are the colon, stomach, female and male organs, the liver, and the lungs. There are some staggering cancer-related statistics. For example, it has been reported that the American Cancer Society estimates that there will be over one million new cases of cancer in 1997, and about 100,000 of that number will represent colon cancer. Most stomach cancer is related to the consumption of products containing caffeine (e.g. commercial teas, coffee, and sodas). Also hundreds of thousands die each year from breast, uterus, prostrate and lung cancer.

Colorectal cancer (in particular) and all other cancers are directly related to constipation and improper activity of eliminative organs (kidney, colon, lungs, and skin). Additionally, the blood system of cancer victims is polluted and toxic. To cure cancer the blood must be detoxified, the eliminative organs must regain vitality, and the immune system must be enhanced.

All natural fruits, vegetables, grains, and quality oils (safflower, sunflower, sesame, etc.) aid in the body's healing. Herbs and herb formulas have been successfully used in treating cancer (e.g. red clover and chaparral, golden seal, pau d'arco and echinacea). Immune strengthening vitamins A, C, and E and minerals magnesium and selenium are important in preventing cancer.

The same herbs and foods that cure cancer also enhance the immune system. In addition to the above-mentioned herbs, ginseng, garlic, dandelion, yellow dock, eucalyptus, and chickweed, aid in building the immune system and curing cancer. Remember, there are very few diseases that cannot be cured with herbs.

Sugar should be avoided since it weakens the immune system. Fresh fruits (alkaline and acid), fresh vegetables, fresh salads, grain, seeds, nuts, sprouts, and beans aid in the healing of all cancers. Specific foods such as barley green, sprouts (especially alfalfa), wheat grass, bee pollen, carrot juice, garlic, lentils, millet, olive oil, and parsley also aid greatly in the healing process.

Most of us eat too many acidic foods which can pollute the blood. Our body needs somewhat of a balance of acid and alkaline foods. Alkaline foods are fruits (cantaloupes, watermelon, honeydews), most vegetables, many grains and legumes. However our saliva will help alkalinize our food if we chew it properly.

The macrobiotic diet and other vegetarian diets has been successfully used in curing cancer and in some cases AIDS. The macrobiotic diet consists of eating whole and fresh foods (fruits, vegetables, grains, legumes, etc.) with very little seasoning. Emphasis is placed on eating fruits and vegetables in the season that they were picked and eating mostly foods grown locally.

Keep in mind cancer (and most other diseases) has a mental and a physical cause. Both must be treated. Emotions must be brought under control. The emotions are the seedbed for cancer. Negative feelings (hatred, anger, resentment, and jealousy) must be sincerely resolved. A greater peace of mind must be achieved.

Whatever the method that one uses to satisfy the above is acceptable as long as it is wholesome. Yoga, exercise, prayer, and mediation are suggestions. Positive thinking and intelligent exercise are effective means of battling cancer on the higher plane.

Most of the time we may need some help. We need supportive, positive people around us. Humor does wonders to quell inner disease. And please don't underestimate the power of a simple hug. They are powerful physical (people) reaffirmations. Get as many as you can.

Become more pleasant about life. Be optimistic even if situations and conditions aren't. Give more intelligently and it will come back in good health and a new view of existence.

Water

The quality of water that we drink has a significant affect on our health condition. Our bodies are mostly masses of water. Our blood is eighty-three percent water, our kidneys eighty-two percent, our muscles seventy-five percent, our brain seventy-four percent, and our bones twenty-two percent.

Water is important in virtually all of the functions of the body. Water is critical to the processes of digestion, elimination, lubrication, regulating temperature, and blood circulation. Pure water also has minerals that are essential to body function.

All the fluids that travel the body are almost all water. For example, the circulatory system (blood), the lymphatic system (lymph fluid), the nervous system (cerebral spinal fluid), the endocrine glands, and the adrenal glands (adrenalin) are vital body systems which are mainly composed of water.

Consuming pure water is essential for optimum health. Consequently, the more balanced and resilient the body is the greater the ability for the inner force within to reach it's potential.

Consider also that all the beverages that we drink whether they are sodas, colas, drinks, vegetable or fruit juices are practically all water. The fruits and vegetables picked from the fields are largely composed of water.

If the water used is not pure we are polluting our body and its systems. And sooner or later it will cause our health condition to depreciate.

Over the years we have consistently polluted our water systems. Factories have dumped all sorts of toxic wastes in the same rivers and streams that we drink from. Municipal water treatment systems use many chemicals to attempt to purify the water. Chlorine, the major chemical in the water-cleaning process is wreaking havoc on our health condition. Chlorine and the other chemicals used in treating water are causing cancers (mainly kidney and bladder cancer), heart attack, stroke, aging, senility and bone diseases.

There are many other potentially health-damaging chemicals in the water that we drink. Some water systems have as many as 100 chemicals in them. Many are very toxic. Ammonia is one example of the type of dangerous additives contained in some drinking water systems.

Most municipal water systems are unfit to drink without a water filter. Spring water is a good alternative, but some springs have been polluted, so be careful. There is some documentation on the water pollution problem. Many studies have been performed on the process of treating drinking water. Generally speaking, larger cities and their environs have more serious drinking water problems.

Those who derive their water from wells or springs should test the water regularly. If it is found to be safe, then it is good quality drinking water.

A large amount of water is used for purposes other than food. Water is used by the millions of gallons in the leather production process, drug and chemical manufacturing, fire protection, and nuclear power plants. Additionally, literally millions of gallons of water are given to animals that are used for consumption (cows, pigs, etc.).

These are not the most expeditious ways to utilize our limited water resources. Water is a precious commodity. Although three-fourths of the earth is water, the great majority of this water cannot be consumed by man and most animals. Therefore, we must always practice water conservation (not just during a drought period). Additionally, we must realize that we can all play a part in wisely using water and our other valuable (and limited) resources.

Why Not Eat (Red) Meat

There are many reasons why we shouldn't eat meat, primarily red meat (e.g. beef and pork). Firstly, meat is the "dead" flesh of an animal and the human digestive system was only meant (or made) to process foods that are "alive". All fruits, vegetables, nuts, grains, or legumes picked from the ground (or vine) are alive and can stay alive and nourish our bodies for a while.

We suffer spiritually from the bad affects of eating the body of animals. When we eat flesh, the spirit of the flesh and the state in which it was slaughtered can adversely effect on our own spiritual being. Eating meat can cause or contribute to increased stress, constipation, obesity, bloated stomach, over emotionalism, mental imbalance, violence, skin problems, cancer, excessive tiredness, heart problems, arthritis, hypertension, osteoporosis, high blood pressure, over aggressiveness and lack of control. White refined sugar causes the same problems. In any case, dis-ease is almost inevitable.

Various forests in North America, Central America, South America (e.g., Brazilian rain forests) and other places are being destroyed for cattle raising, thereby, eliminating the most valuable means of reversing the ozone layer depletion. Meat production greatly contributes to water pollution. Animals consume lots of water.

It takes more than 2500 gallons of water to produce 1 pound of meat. Ironically it takes 20 gallons of water to yield one pound of wheat. In fact livestock production accounts for almost half of the water consumed in America.

If you are looking for more incentives to cease or greatly reduce your meat intake, consider this. The average grown meat eater has about a 50% chance of heart attack. Meanwhile the average pure vegetarian has less than a 5% chance of heart attack. Consider also if Americans would reduce their meat intake by 10% we would save enough grains to fed the 60 million people worldwide who starve to death each year.

The statistics from this section were excerpted from the book *"Diet for a New America"* by John Robbins. This book explains even more of the ill effects of eating meat.

Our Health Status

"Give a man a fish he will live for a day, teach a man to fish he will live forever."

A Children's World view

This is one of the most important sections of this writing. For we perpetuate disease, ill-health, and related adversities through our children. We perpetuate thoughts, dispositions, values, and attitudes through young people.

Habits, good or bad are usually started young. So why not emphasize the good and train our children when young to practice good nutrition habits? It is an investment that will pay off later.

The first bit of advice for expecting mothers or breast-feeding mothers is to improve your diet. What you eat your baby eats too. Eat plenty of fresh fruits and vegetables, nuts, seeds, and juices. Fresh fruit juice (e.g. oranges or lemons diluted in water), or vegetable juice (e.g. carrot, beet, or cucumber) are good. Lemons are full of vitamin C. Carrot juice should be the preferred beverage because it has so many nutrients and it is normally sweet tasting (one eight-ounce glass is sufficient).

Babies and Younger Children

Very young children need the proper environment and nourishment to grow. The foods that they eat influence how much and how fast they grow. Vitamins, minerals, proteins, carbohydrates, and fats must be present in proper amounts for balanced mental and physical growth.

There are certain rules that if followed will assure success. First read books and articles that discuss the nutritional needs of young children. Then identify a doctor, herbalist, nutritional advisor, or others with whom you can consult.

You do not have to feed your child cow's milk or dairy products. There are many other foods that will provide the nutrients that these food supplies and without side effects (e.g., mucous). Cow milk contains casein. Casein helps in the development of bones. It is in much greater concentration in cow's milk than breast milk. It can be easily digested by cows but not by humans. It forms undigested curds in the stomach. Thus it is just another toxin in the body that is difficult to eliminate. Also casein is a major ingredient in the manufacture of wood glue, so you can understand that it has no place in the body (in large amounts).

Mother's milk is far superior to cow's milk. Even a mother with a bad diet should breast-feed her child but add to her diet the proper nutrients. Cow's milk is for cows. It tends to cause the baby's body to grow faster physically than mentally. Initially a human should grow faster mentally and calves should grow faster physically.

Proper nutrition is necessary for children. Calcium, protein, and the vitamins A, E, B and C are important to the proper growth in children. There are foods that contain many of these nutrients. Green vegetables (e.g. kale, spinach, or collards greens) and fruits (e.g. lemons, apples, or grapes) are examples.

Carrots, soy products, fruits, wheat products and other grains have most of the necessary nutrients. And yes, you can get both calcium and protein from fruits, vegetables, grains, legumes, and seeds. By combining non-meat sources intelligently such as grains (whole wheat bread) and legumes (peanut butter) you will get all eight essential amino acids of protein.

Soy and tofu (made from soy) products are very good alternatives to dairy products. They are health-giving natural foods rich in vitamins and minerals. They are the backbone of a meatless diet, free of chemical toxins and low in cost. Both are easy to digest and very low in calories. They can be used to make great tasting beverages, desserts, cheese, meatless entrees and appetizers.

Soy milk possesses most of the essential amino acids of protein and has more calcium than cow's milk. Other essential vitamins and minerals are also present in soy milk and soy products. Nut milk (e.g., almond milk) is another good source of protein and calcium without much mucous.

Mother's milk is a balanced nutritious meal. Mother's milk has a sufficient amount of vitamins, minerals, proteins, and enzymes for the baby's nourishment. But a mother must consistently eat nutritious food and take food additives (e.g., herbs and other supplements) for the child to receive maximum nutrition.

Mothers should breast-feed their children for at least six months but not more than two years. One year is a typical period of time before the baby is weaned off of breast milk. Then feed the child unprocessed, unchemicalized baby food with no sugar (e.g. peas, carrots, squash, sweet potatoes) and definitely no animal products. You may also feed your baby food that is blended, mashed or cut into small pieces since the baby cannot effectively chew food. Gradually you may introduce the child to table food but make the food simple. Babies love fruit (e.g. bananas) blended or mashed. Fruit makes a great nutritious meal. Fruit and vegetable juices are excellent for babies. They have many of the necessary nutrients for growth in the form that a baby can easily use.

Carrot juice whether by itself or mixed with beet, celery, cucumber, or other juices has great amounts of nutrients (e.g. Vitamins A, B, C, E, proteins, calcium and other minerals) and taste good. Don't mix fruit and vegetable juices. Use a balance of acid (oranges, lemons, and grapefruit), subacid (dates, bananas, cherries, grapes, apples, etc.) and alkaline fruits (cantaloupe, watermelon, and honeydew).

Oatmeal and oats are an excellent food for babies and adults. They possess high amounts of calcium, B- vitamins, and protein. Green vegetables are very good too since they contain calcium, minerals, and protein.

Tofu and tempeh are good meat substitutes. They have protein, calcium, and other nutrients. Rice, beans, and most wheat products are good too. But over consumption of grains and soya products can produce excess mucous especially in children. Although this mucous is not the same (and not as harmful to the body) as the mucous obtained from meats and dairy products, it can still cause problems (e.g. colds or runny nose). But if you eat these foods properly you shouldn't have a mucous problem.

You should make sure that you combine your grains and legumes properly (e.g. rice and beans, peanut butter and breads) so that you get all 8 essential amino acids of protein. Keep in mind that if you eat enough grains, legumes, fruits, and vegetables, you get your complete protein requirements. In fact, the average vegetarian gets 150% of the daily protein requirement.

A word of caution about dairy products. They are not as healthy as certain organizations (e.g. Milk Marketing Board) suggest. Dairy products (and an impacted, waste-filled colon) are the main cause of most childhood diseases (mumps, measles, chicken pox, flu, etc.). Milk of course is the main contributor. Cows are given many drugs to help them grow faster, have leaner meat, and weight more.

Many cows feed on food that has been sprayed with dangerous pesticides (e.g. dioxin, PCB's). These chemicals go into the milk. Baby formulas are not much better than cow's milk. Goat's milk is a good source of nutrition containing calcium, phosphorus and vitamin D. But the other problem with milk is the high cholesterol and fat content. Also many people have a problem digesting milk.

Milk, cheese, and eggs are high fat and high cholesterol foods. They can cause a variety of health problems. But eggs eaten sparingly (e.g. 2 or 3 times weekly) may be satisfactory for those in transition. Eggs contain many essential vitamins and minerals and possess all of the essential amino acids of protein. And for those vegetarians who are worried about an adequate amount of B-12, eggs are a better option than other animal foods.

Don't feed young children sugar (white refined) or any products with sugar in them (e.g. cakes, cookies, ice cream, candy, donuts or sodas). Don't train a child's taste buds to prefer such a dangerous addictive substance. Use natural sweets (e.g. maple syrup, grain sweeteners or pure honey as a substitute. Children under one year of age shouldn't eat honey but instead can have maple syrup. There are several companies who make excellent tasting, naturally sweetened fruit juice beverages, and all natural desserts.

Don't feed your children red meat (beef or pork). If you want to feed them chicken and fish do so only when they are old enough to chew properly. If your children are hyperactive it's probably because they have parasites in them. Parasites grow and multiply when we eat sugar, animal products, and white flour products. They cannot survive in a body where whole foods and herbs are consumed.

Don't give your children drugs (legal or illegal). If they get sick use herbal or homeopathic remedies. If there is absolutely no other option (in most cases there are) use medicines, but only for a short time. Remember if your child eats as we have recommended all sicknesses will be minor and manageable. The herb echinacea is good for colds, flu, tonsillitis, fever, insect bites, and excess mucous.

Vaccinations are very questionable ways of preventing contagious diseases. There can be an element of danger in vaccinations in that they can cause sickness, cancer, and even death. Also many children and adults have become crippled by the polio, smallpox, flu, diphtheria, typhoid, and other vaccinations. Most vaccinations damage the immune system. Most people are not aware of the fact that in the typical vaccination a sample of the actual disease is used.

Generally speaking vaccinations are dangerous. If you disbelieve this just ask your doctor to give you a written, certified guarantee assuring you of the safety of the vaccination. He won't.

In most states one is within their constitutional and religious rights to refuse any vaccinations. In many states you only have to sign a form releasing the authorities from responsibility (legally). Also, consult with a doctor or other health professional who is aware of the options and alternatives. If you do get yourself or your children vaccinated and you're concerned about health ramifications, take immune strengthening herbs (e.g. echinacea, panl d'arco, or garlic).

There are many great tasting and nutritious foods for young children. Check with your local health food store. You will find many good packaged foods. Whether you shop in the health food store or supermarket, read labels and don't forget fresh fruits. Remember that your child is your responsibility and you must do your best to give them the healthiest start in life.

Older Children and Young Adults

Most teenagers have deplorable diets. The high paced, commercialized fast food lifestyle will eventually cause all sorts of health problems. The gall bladder, kidney, appendix, heart, brain, and the lungs are some of the problem areas affected by reckless and irresponsible dietary habits.

Too many of our children have health problems attributed to the over- consumption of fat by age 21. Most parents don't know enough and don't take enough time to monitor their child's diets. Processed foods and microwave foods make up the bulk of children's diet.

Food advertisers promote great tasting foods that have little nutritive value. School lunches are as much as fifty percent fat. Many children are hooked on junk foods. Sodas, cereals, processed fast food, and potato chips supply their food requirements. These foods are laden with sugar, salt, and/or chemical additives. For example, hamburgers, french fries, and steaks are more than fifty percent fat. Most breakfast cereals and candies are fifty to eighty percent sugar.

These foods cause all the common health problems that adults have. Children should be trained to read labels, comprehend ingredients, and not eat bad foods. They should know what kinds of problems may occur if they eat junk foods. For example, potato chips help make cavities. Sugar causes hyperactivity, pre-diabetic and diabetic problems, laziness, appendix and gall bladder problems. And high fat foods lead to weight problems. Additionally, these foods cause constipation, circulatory problems, mental maladies, and eventually serious disease.

Children and teenagers should eat fresh fruits and vegetables. Whole grains legumes, and unroasted nuts are also important. Homemade soups and/or fresh salads should be prepared daily. Most children should take a multivitamin and mineral supplement. This will insure that they will get the basic requirements. However, you cannot eat bad food and take vitamins while expecting good health. Adolescents and children should take certain herbs in order to maintain good health such as: comfrey (calcium), echinacea (general cleanser), garlic (blood and heart), and senna (constipation).

Remember peer pressure is tremendous. Other children, whose parents don't know (or don't care) about proper dietary habits may taunt and ridicule your children. To resolve this you must explain to your children why they eat differently. Then take them to see some sick people in a hospital or nursing home. Tell them that a lot of their uninformed friends will also be sick and ill when they grow older. That is if their diet doesn't cause their demise first.

Health Concerns for Males and Females

It is important for women and men to be more concerned with proper nutrition and healthy foods in their young adult years. Their bodies can be vulnerable to health problems at any age. Women are usually more concerned with their bodies. Therefore women tend to go to the doctor more frequently than men.

Two of the areas which tend to be affected the most by health maladies in females are the uterus and the breast. The numbers of females who have breast and uterine cancer as well as fibroid tumors and related problems are great.

Additionally osteoporosis (loss of bone mass) is more than twice as likely to affect women than men. One out of four women have complications related to osteoporosis and many people with osteoporosis die of falls and accidents where critical bones are broken.

Although the process of giving birth is a natural process (usually without complications), difficulties can occur if proper dietary habits are not followed. Caesarean sections become likely because of poor diet and lack of exercise (in most instances). Most babies that are born with defects, stillborn, or who are victims of miscarriage are the result of a poor diet that provides very few nutrients to the mother and the baby inside of her. Drugs, tobacco, and alcohol are substances that can also cause pregnancy-related problems. A pregnant woman eats for herself and her baby. Additionally, if a pregnant woman is under emotional stress and doesn't take the proper nutrients, those emotions can directly affect the baby inside of her.

Contrary to popular belief the great majority of all hysterectomies, mastectomies, and C-sections are unnecessary. There is some documentation in the medical reports and journals to substantiate this. If you are a possible candidate for any of these medical procedures, you must immediately go on a nutrition and herb program. Be sure to find a trained health practitioner who is familiar with herbs and nutritional healing (herbalist, doctor, chiropractor, or others). Also, do your own research.

For most problems the answer is the same. Go on a whole foods diet with plenty of raw fruits and vegetables. Take herbs for calcium (comfrey), colon cleansing (senna, cascara sagrada, or aloe), blood cleanser (burdock, echinacea, chaparral, or dandelion) and immune system enhancement (e.g. rose hips, fresh garlic, echinacea, paul d'arco or golden seal).

Males should be more concerned with their health. For traditionally males have paid little attention to their health until signs of problems are manifested. Pain is usually the signal that brings attention to health problems for men. In most instances, by the time we get pain, the problem has ensued for too long.

Prostrate problems are increasing rapidly. More than ten percent of all men have prostrate problems. The American Cancer Society estimates that one out of eleven males will get prostrate cancer and that it is the second leading cause of cancer death in men. A bad diet is the main cause but there are other contributing factors such as prostrate-related infections. Also older men have the greatest risk of getting prostrate cancer.

While alcohol and cigarettes affect everyone, males are victimized more by lung cancer (smoking) and liver problems (alcohol). It has been reported that the American Lung Association estimates that males have eighty percent more lung cancer, and that lung cancer is the number one form of cancer. Males are slightly ahead of females on alcohol-related liver problems. Both habits pollute the blood, damage the immune system and the liver. These habits also adversely affect our energy level. The lungs' ability to get oxygen to the blood and eliminate waste is impaired by smoking. Alcohol has an adverse affect on digestion and in time will destroy the liver.

Improper foods have a deleterious affect on the eliminative organs of both males and females. Waste or mucous (by-products of bad foods or improperly digested foods) gathers around all the eliminative organs. This waste wants to get out and tries to leave the body in the normal way. However, large amounts of it doesn't leave the body.

The prostrate (in the male) and the uterus (in the female) are collectors of this waste. The breasts are also areas where this waste collects. And consequently these are the areas where health problems can occur frequently. Prostrate problems (including impotency, prostrate cancer, inability to reproduce) are related to this buildup of waste. The American Cancer Society estimates that there will be 334,500 new cases of prostrate cancer and 180,200 new cases of breast cancer in 1997.

Fibroid tumors, ovary problems, pregnancy-related difficulties, and imbalances in hormones are all related to this accumulation of waste in the body. All infections as well as most sexually transmitted diseases are related to this buildup of waste. In fact, most hysterectomies are related to this waste.

Candida albicans, which is another disease that affects mainly women, is related to this waste buildup. It is a common yeast like fungus which can be found in or on almost everyone. When we are in good health, our natural body defenses can keep it under control. Otherwise it can multiply quickly and cause many health problems, such as skin and menstrual problems, white vaginal discharge, colic, and asthma.

Rebuilding the immune system and clearing the waste out of the body will aid in alleviating all of these problems. There are certain herbs that help get rid of waste in the genital areas. Red raspberry (for females) and golden seal (for males) are two of the more used herbs. Golden seal is a powerful cleanser of the entire body. Acidophilus has also been used to treat candida.

Constipation and an impacted colon (a putrefied, waste-filled colon) are contributing factors to all problems related to the uterus. The colon is located above the uterus. When it becomes impacted, it loses it's normal shape (which is an upside down U) and eventually it will press down on the uterus. Many hysterectomies are performed where the real problem is an impacted colon. Although slow, irregular bowels is the first sign of an impacted colon, there are others. Excessive mucous, low energy, a bloated stomach are other likely signs.

But overall body toxicity is the main problem. Even a woman's menstrual cycle is related to this. The woman's monthly cycle (period) is just a woman's body ridding itself of toxins. Generally, the longer the period, the more polluted the body is. In a fairly healthy body, the period should not last longer than three days.

There are women from remote areas and tropical islands who have periods of four hours or less (with a light flow). These women eat mostly raw fruits and vegetables and drink pure water. They also have less stressful lives and do not have sex frequently which are two other factors in reducing body toxicity and a woman's monthly cycle.

Additionally, women who exercise have a decreased monthly cycle. The main reason why is that exercise and sweating will rid the body of toxins. And the body has less toxins to get rid of through menstruation. Hence, the period is shorter. Red raspberry shortens the period, eliminate cramps, and clean and tones the uterus.

The Overly Seasoned Citizens: Our Seniors

Most of our seasoned citizens are sick, in pain, or have several health problems as the result of the cumulative affects of bad dietary habits. Even people in their thirties, forties, and fifties are afflicted with similar illnesses.

Cancer, heart attacks, stroke, diabetes, arthritis, and many more illnesses are common among older people. And today the middle-aged are experiencing similar problems. It's not all their fault, since the knowledge was not as replete as it is today. But Mother Nature doesn't care if you know or not.

About forty million Americans have arthritis. Arthritis is the result of damage to the bone cartilage. It is characterized by joint inflammation, pain, swelling, stiffness, and restricted mobility. The cause is the same as previously mentioned, namely, a bad diet, specifically the over-consumption of meats (beef and pork) as well as dairy products and sugar. Meats have uric acid that build up in the body to eventually cause arthritis, rheumatism and/or gout.

Doctors make millions of dollars on seasoned citizens' illnesses and the cost is absorbed by private insurance or a government health plan. The cost of traditional medical health care is on the increase. A one week hospital stay typically costs between $30,000 and $40,000 and that's steadily increasing. Dr. C. Everett Koop (the former surgeon General) once said, and I paraphrase, "there is something wrong with a system (medical delivery system) that requires more and more money to service fewer people."

A large number of Americans are getting older. Within the next ten years or so the baby boom generation will be approaching over fifty. And they will get sicker because of a high fat, high protein, acid-producing diet.

Older people are the most likely victims of the medical and drug industries' mistakes and negligence in pursuit of profit. The seniors are many times given overdoses of drugs and in some cases unneeded drugs or drugs that don't address the immediate health problem.

More than seventy thousand seniors die each year because of the prescribing of wrong medicines (drugs). Mistakes in prescribing drugs are much more common than we realize. And the problem is getting worse. Also keep in mind that in the majority of senior deaths, there is no autopsy performed to determine if drugs were related to their deaths.

Additionally, the drug companies, which usually are part of huge multi-billion dollar corporate structures, offer free gifts and vacations to doctors for prescribing a particular new medicine or medicines. In many instances the doctors don't know the full story on the possible side-effects of these drugs. In the future our seniors may even be more victimized unless controls and regulations are instituted.

Unfortunately, most seasoned citizens experience bad health more often than they experience good health. The cumulative affects of bad eating have set in. Everyday becomes a greater burden. They don't walk as fast and they don't think as fast. They also have a harder time taking care of themselves. It doesn't have to be that way in most cases. The best advise is to take dietary precautions when you are young. Then in your older years, your state of health will be at least fair.

Senility and aging are related to diet. There are many people in the world who live to be over 100 years old in good health. The oldest known person in the world in modern time lived in China and was well over 200 years old. The eldest documented person lived in Japan and was 120 years old.

Remember age causes no disease. Only cumulative violations of our bodies cause disease. Eating quality foods (very few processed foods and animal products) and taking the previously mentioned herbs (burdock, echinacea, comfrey, etc.) will slow the aging process. Stress and worry also accelerate the aging process. So don't get too upset. If you do, just eat right and take extra herbs and vitamins.

Meats, dairy products, sugar, excess protein, and white flour products accelerate the aging process. So does caffeine, drugs, tobacco, and alcohol. And all the above leech (take) calcium out of the body. All the former contribute to rheumatism, arthritis, osteoporosis, and other ailments.

All the above bad food and habits must be eliminated. Herbs, natural foods, and right thinking are a must. Older people require more care and concern than others. It is good for them to associate with people and remain active.

Vitamins A, E and C and the minerals selenium and zinc are potent antioxidants, which strengthen the immune system and help reverse the aging process. Calcium is also important for older people. Calcium strengthens the bones and all body organs. It will help eliminate arthritis, rheumatism, and osteoporosis. It should be taken as an herb supplement (rose hips, comfrey, or alfalfa) or taken in the many non-animal foods (oats, oatmeal, soy milk, tofu, sesame seeds, seaweed, etc.). However the herbs guarantee that one gets an ample supply of these nutrients.

Burdock, which is a very good blood purifier, helps reduce swellings and deposits in the joints in arthritis. Alfalfa and yucca reduces inflammation in the joints. Herbs, fasting, and cleansing the colon with enemas may reduce pain. Alfalfa has a great combination of vitamins and minerals as well as possessing the eight-essential amino acids of protein. Chaparral, burdock, alfalfa, and a very mild colon cleanser (those already mentioned) used together will help the previously mentioned diseases that afflict many seasoned citizens in most cases.

The non-animal calcium sources should be combined with a vitamin D source since vitamin D helps the body absorb calcium. Also the sun's ultraviolet rays help our body to make some amount of vitamin D but the sun must be supplemented with vitamin D in foods and/or herbs.

Our seasoned citizens should remain active and productive in many ways. Community involvement is a viable means of staying active. Working with the young is also a great benefit to our seniors. Also seniors should socialize with each other.

Exercise helps the body absorb calcium more effectively. Seniors should exercise as much as possible. Simple walking is a good exercise. Many of the exercises that young people do, seniors can do as well. Attitude is an important ingredient. Keep the spirits high.

The Good

"The doctor of the future will give no medicine but will interest his patients in the care of the human frame and in the cause and prevention of disease." Thomas Edison

Doing the Right Things

Most people think that they are giving up personal rights when you suggest that they alter their eating habits. It is not easy to change bad eating habits but the rewards are priceless, namely, life and health. Greater energy, increased mental capacity, and a more radiant appearance are also the rewards of good eating habits. Good eating habits also help one to be more at peace and less emotional.

Just like bad habits, we can train our minds into good habits. One of the methods is gradually make small dietary changes. For good food is the chief ingredient in and the cornerstone of proper nutrition. So be consistent, persistent and keep making changes until you get all the bad foods out of your diet.

The foods to eliminate in order to be healthy are: white sugar, meat, and white flour products. Also you must reduce the amount of dairy products, salt, and processed, chemicalized foods that you eat. It is also important to decrease the amount of food eaten on a daily basis. Eating a lot of food doesn't mean that you are healthy. One should eat to nourish the body's cells. That can only be done by eating a good quality of foods not a good quantity.

Proteins

Foods can be broken down into protein, carbohydrates, and fats. Proteins are food substances necessary to build and rebuild strong healthy tissue. Every organ and tissue in the body is composed of protein. Proteins are composed of amino acids. There are twenty two amino acids. All but eight can be made by the body.

These eight are; isoleucine, leucine, lysine, methane, phenylalanine, tryptophan, threonine, and valine.

Proteins are derived from foods and food supplements in the diet. A complete protein has all the eight amino acids. Few good, quality foods are complete proteins. Soy products such as soybeans, tofu, soy milk contain most of the amino acids of proteins. We can get complete protein from other natural foods normally by combining certain incomplete protein food sources. The best food sources to combine are legumes and grains, for example brown rice and beans, peanut butter and bread, corn bread and black-eyed peas, etc. By eating whole grains, fruits, vegetables and legumes (e.g. nuts, beans, black-eye peas) a vegetarian gets plenty of protein.

There are many natural foods which are a good source of protein such as salad greens, nuts, grains, potatoes, and most vegetables. If you want to eat a good animal source of protein, the only foods I would recommend are: eggs, fish (e.g. bluefish, whiting, bass, porgies, and other scaled fish with bones) or fowl (e.g. turkey or chicken).

Eggs are the best quality protein of all the animal products. Chicken and fish are better protein sources than other flesh. But they should be baked, boiled, broiled, or roasted. Yogurt is another complete protein source. But there is too much sugar and dairy products in most supermarket yogurts.

There is one company that makes a tofu (instead of milk) based yogurt with honey (instead of sugar). Certain herbs such as alfalfa and spirulina are very good protein sources. Also most of the herbs with lots of protein have many other valuable nutrients.

But remember you do not need as much protein as many conventional dieticians and nutritionists may suggest. We only need about fifty grams of protein per day (about ten percent of our total calories). In fact, too much animal protein is the cause of many health maladies (e.g. heart problems, arthritis, cancer, sinus, constipation). Additionally we could eat one food from the "nut" group and one from the "grain" group in small quantities and have enough protein for the day. Also too much animal protein causes calcium to be leeched from the body.

The average vegetarian consumes fifty percent more protein than the recommended daily allowance which is more than sufficient. Additionally, the quality of protein that vegetarians eat is a better quality than non-vegetarians and is more easily absorbed and assimilated by the body.

An elephant gets all the necessary protein in one peanut and a few other foods like alfalfa in one day. Cows weigh a few thousand pounds, and eat mostly grass and herbs like alfalfa and dandelion. Most animals in the wild don't eat meat, and they are big and strong. Perhaps they are more intelligent or have not abandoned good common sense and intelligence for technological advancement. Not that technological advancement is bad. It just can't replace or enhance (completely) what Mother Nature has designed. Additionally, you do not have to eat the foods that provide you with all essential amino acids at each meal.

Carbohydrates and Fats

Carbohydrates are composed of the chemical elements carbon, hydrogen, and oxygen with the latter two being in the same proportion as water (H_2O). The various starches and sugars are the carbohydrates which provide nourishment in our foods. The simple sugars which are glucose, fructose, and galactose. Complex carbohydrates (the union of simple sugars) must be broken down into simple sugars.

Carbohydrates provide energy (fuel) to the body. They also allow the body to make some B-vitamins and are part of the structure of many biological compounds. Carbohydrates can be produced cheaply in abundance. They provide Americans with thirty to fifty percent of their food energy. They should provide fifty to eighty percent of our food energy.

Carbohydrates include the following: wheat, rice, corn, oats, potatoes, many fruits and vegetables, peas, beans, sugar cane, honey, beets, and many processed foods (jams, jellies, molasses, noodles, spaghetti, dried fruits, breads and other baked goods).

Starch is an important carbohydrate food source. Through digestion the body changes the starch in foods to glucose, which can be used as a source of energy by the body. If the body receives more glucose than it can use as energy, some of it can be stored as glycogen in the liver and muscle tissues. But carbohydrates consumed in excess are rapidly converted to fat. This is the chief way of becoming overweight. The excess food becomes waste (unusable food) in the body.

Fats are another food necessary for body function. Fats are composed of fatty acids (oils) and glycerol. Unsaturated and polyunsaturated fatty acids are better quality and healthier than saturated fatty acids. Eating too many foods high in saturated fats can cause health problems (e.g. heart, blood, constipation, etc.).

All food fats, animal or vegetable contain a mixture of saturated and unsaturated fatty acids. Animal fats are much more saturated than vegetable fats and oils made from animal fats are much more saturated than vegetable oils. Coconut oil (one of the exceptions) is highly saturated as is beef and chocolate. In fact, beef has a much higher percentage of fatty acids than fish or chicken.

There are many unsaturated fat foods in the oil form. Safflower, corn, sesame, cottonseed,sunflower, peanut, and soybean oils are unsaturated and are rich in linoleic acid (an essential fatty acid necessary in small amounts for growth and healthy skin). Fats are also necessary for reproduction, lubrication, utilization of the fat soluble vitamins A, D, E, and K, and provide a concentrated source of energy.

Many foods have two or all of the basic food elements. The best form to get the nutritional needs for the body is in natural foods cooked without preservatives or additives, and containing no sugar.

Vitamins

Vitamins are vital to the proper functioning of the body. The prefix for the word vitamin is "vita" which means life. Vitamins enhance the cells and rejuvenate the body. Vitamins and minerals in supplements can be a very useful tool in nutrifying the body.

There are two types of vitamins, namely, fat soluble and water soluble. The fat soluble vitamins (A, D, E, and K) were previously mentioned as being absorbed with fat. Without a sufficient amount of good quality oils (fats), these vitamins cannot be effectively absorbed, hence a vitamin deficiency may result. However, these vitamins can be easily stored in the body for a period of time.

Water soluble vitamins (B-complex and C) must be replaced in the body daily since they are excreted out the body and cannot be stored. These are also the most important vitamins although they are all important.

Vitamin C is the most important vitamin. It is important for so many body functions and is essential for many metabolic processes. It is important in the breakdown of protein and in maintaining a high energy level. It helps to heal fractures and wounds. It helps the body absorb iron and is a powerful antioxidant (attacks free radicals which cause cancer). It is a well known cold remedy.

Vitamin C helps strengthen the immune system, which is the key to maintaining good health and fighting off body toxins. A strong immune system enhances our body's ability to fight diseases like cancer and AIDS.

Vitamin C is also important to the formation of collagen which holds the cells together.

Vitamin C calms the nerves and reduces stress. It aids in healing mental problems, arthritis, infections, drug problems, sinus, and heart maladies. There has been research completed by the medical community on the effectiveness of vitamin C in treating cancer, heart, and other problems.

Taking high doses of vitamin C as well as the immune strengthening herbs (e.g. paul d'arco, garlic, golden seal and echinacea) is an effective way of arresting and eliminating many chronic and terminal ailments. Many foods and herbs have good amounts of vitamin C.

The best form to take vitamin C is the herb rose hips because it is a natural herb. Other forms such as ascorbic acid are manufactured from rose hips. Rose hips also contains vitamin E, A, D, and collagen, an antiwrinkling agent. It also contains most of the B-complex vitamins as well as having significant amounts of calcium and iron. Many foods have good amounts of this vitamin such as carrots, greens, parsley, cabbage, broccoli, strawberries, and citrus fruit.

The B-vitamins provide energy to the body. They aid in the functioning of the brain, the nerves, and the body's metabolism of nutrients. There are 11 elements in the B-complex family and all are important. They are B-1 (thiamine), B-2 (riboflavin), niacin, B-6 (pyridoxine), B-12, pantothenic acid, PABA, biotin, choline, inositol, and folic acid. They should be taken as a group.

The B-vitamins are valuable under stress. Pantothenic acid is very good for stress. The vitamin B-1 is related to mental health and learning capacity. The vitamin B-2 may help with personality problems. The vitamin B-3 helps relieve depression. The vitamin B-6 helps metabolize tryptophan, which is an essential amino acid that helps calm the body. Vitamin B-12 prevents anemia, as well as nervous and psychological disorders (e.g. paranoia). Other than energy and nerves the B-vitamins aid in the metabolism of carbohydrates, amino acids, and fatty acids.

Vegetarians have to be concerned with their B-12 intake since this vitamin is not widely found in non-meat food sources. A B-12 deficiency can result in central nervous system damage and mental abnormalities. A B-6 deficiency may result in depression, irritability, skin irritations, and intestinal problems.

Foods that have a good amount of the B-complex vitamins are whole grains, whole cereals, dark green, leafy vegetables, wheat germ, brewer's yeast, eggs and carob (chocolate substitute). It is probably good to take a B-complex supplement to be sure we have enough.

Bulghar wheat has a good amount of B-vitamins. The herbs cholorella, bee pollen, ginkgo, alfalfa, spirulina, gota kola, parsley, passion flower, and eyebright also have good amounts of B-vitamins. All have B-12 in considerable amounts. The herbs which help the brain and the head contain the B-complex vitamins. Eggs, fish, and liver have a good amount of all the B-vitamins.

Echinacea, alfalfa, comfrey, dandelion and several other herbs have considerable amounts of vitamin A. Vitamin A is important to the skin, eyes, the digestive and respiratory systems. It is a valuable antioxidant. Antioxidants protect the body from cellular breakdown. They (antioxidants) retain free radicals, which are environmental toxins (e.g. pesticides, air and water pollution), that attack the immune system and speed up the aging process. Sources of vitamin A are sweet potatoes, squash, carrots, and eggs. One should not take doses of vitamin A in excess because it can be dangerous.

Beta carotene also called pro-vitamin A is converted in the body to vitamin A. It is a better supplemental form of vitamin A. Research has been completed on beta carotene's positive affect on the immune system and cancer. Carrots, yams, and some green vegetables contain beta carotene.

Vitamin E is an antioxidant and together with vitamin C slows down the aging process. It prevents blood clotting and helps prevent heart attacks, strokes, and related problems. Vegetable oils are a good source of vitamin E. Burdock, blue cohosh, angelica, bee pollen, and echinacea also have good amounts of vitamin E.

Vitamin D is essential for the absorption of calcium. Calcium helps us to maintain strong bones. The body can make vitamin D from the ultraviolet light of the sun. So a little sunshine can help your calcium go a long way. The herbs barberry, dandelion, alfalfa, and most herbs that help the liver contain vitamin D.

Vitamin K can be manufactured by the body for the most part. It is important for blood clotting and the normal function of the liver. Green leafy vegetables, tomatoes, and eggs are sources of vitamin K. Cornsilk, gota kola, safflower, slippery elm, and other herbs have this vitamin.

Minerals

Minerals are a very important and needed ingredient in body health. There are 103 known minerals and all plants, animals and humans need various ones. We must consume them regularly because they are easily excreted out of the body.

Calcium, phosphorus, magnesium, sodium, potassium, sulfur, and silicon are the regular minerals, The trace minerals are iron, manganese, chromium, zinc, copper, cobalt, molybdenum, fluorine, iodine, selenium, vanadium, and gold.

Calcium is the most important mineral. It aids in the development of bone and tissue. It is important in the development of teeth and organ tissue (e.g. heart, lungs, brain, etc.). It helps the blood to clot and aids in enhancing vitality and endurance. It contributes more to bone density than any other nutrient. Without it bones become weak, brittle, and porous, therefore become susceptible to fracture.

Soy milk, tofu, soybeans, green vegetables, oats, oatmeal, carrots, bulghar wheat, carob, and many grains have good amounts of calcium. The herbs comfrey, dandelion, camomile, peppermint, horsetail, cayenne, rose hips, kelp, yellow dock, plantain and alfalfa have calcium and other nutrients. As was previously stated, we need vitamin D for calcium to effectively do its job.

Phosphorus plays an important role in the growth of bones and tissue. It also helps our bodies metabolize carbohydrates, proteins, and fats. Zinc improves the body's ability to fight off disease. Insufficient amounts of it can offset weight loss, inhibit growth and sexual development, cause hair loss, and have an adverse affect on the skin, the eyes, the healing of wounds, and the appetite.

The minerals selenium and zinc are antioxidants that have a positive effect on the immune system and slow the aging process. Studies have substantiated zinc's ability to restore the immune function. Selenium neutralizes the adverse affects of toxins. Zinc shouldn't be taken in large doses.

Germanium has a positive affect on the immune system. Magnesium helps build healthy nerves and muscles. Chromium aids fat and sugar metabolism and hence strengthens the heart. Iron prevents anemia. Potassium is an essential factor in blood building. Potassium controls the activity of the heart, muscles, the nervous system, kidneys, and muscle tone. It aids in the growth process for children.

Copper is important in the formation of red blood cells and in skeletal development. It is also necessary for the absorption and utilization of iron. Cobalt maintains red blood cells and functions as a part of B-12. It is also necessary for normal growth.

Iodine regulates energy production and the rate of metabolism. It is good for the skin, hair, nails, and teeth. The herbs alfalfa and kelp contain the great majority of minerals and what mineral alfalfa doesn't have kelp has. Alfalfa and kelp are also good vitamin sources.

Herbs

Herbs are the key to good health and a stable mind. Herbs are live plants, trees, vines, etc. that give life and renew the life force within us. Every food that grows is an herb. Apples, strawberries, potatoes, corn, avocado, etc. are all herbs. Herbs can also be used for cooking (e.g. cloves, cinnamon, nutmeg, and parsley) and for aromatic (scents) purposes. Aromatic herbs can be used to relax and soothe (e.g. eucalyptus or lavender) or to inspire (e.g. rosemary). They can also be used in massage therapy (e.g. spearmint) or can be used to create an atmosphere of serenity (e.g. orange blossom) or sensuality (e.g. rose).

The herbs we are concentrating on are those used for medicinal purposes. They are still foods. In fact the FDA classifies herbs not as drugs, but as foods.

There are over 600,000 herbs throughout the world. Less than 600 are poisonous. They have very few side affects. They are natural as is for the body. And nature works best in the natural.

Herbs are referred to in the Bible in many places such as: *Ezekiel* 47:12; *Genesis* 9:3; *Psalms* 104:35; I *Corinthians* 3:7-8; *Jeremias* 12:4 and *Proverbs* 15:17. They were used for their curative powers but also for other purposes. Aloe which heals and energizes the body is mentioned frequently. Mint which cools and calms the body is mentioned in *Matthew* 23:23. Camomile, comfrey, garlic, parsley, and others are mentioned.

Herbs have been used since the beginning of time for food, rejuvenation, and illnesses. In previous times most people had some knowledge of herbs. In fact many older people from the southern parts of the country still use herbs. And in the future it may be mandatory that most people have at least a limited knowledge of herbs.

Wholistic healing is one of the main facets of herbs. Herbs seek to heal the problem instead of just the symptom. For example, if you have a bad cold, the herbs will not only alleviate the sneezing, coughing, or running nose but will also help to eliminate the mucous (waste) out of the system, which is the real problem.

Herbs can stimulate body organs and work with the body to promote healing. And they do so in accord with nature, not like drugs which work against nature to treat symptoms. No doctor, engineer or chemist can duplicate what Mother Nature has produced. Herbs work with Mother Nature to enhance life.

For every condition or ailment that you can think of there is an herb that will aid in the cure. By no means is that a bold statement. There are several herb books available in health food stores. There are millions of people in the world with a knowledge of herbs and hundreds of thousands who are herbalists. There are probably a few who live in the general vicinity where you are.

Herbal knowledge may not be considered important by most Americans but more Americans are becoming aware of the significance of herbs. Besides the fact that the foods we eat that come from the earth are herbs, every vitamin comes from an herb. Almost every drug has an herb in it and herbs are the foods that most animals eat.

Herbs can be taken in several forms. Teas, capsules and caplets are the main forms in which herbs are taken. They can also be taken in the form of extracts which are herb powders that are liquefied.

In the past, scientists and chemists extract one ingredient out of an herb to make a vitamin or a drug, when that herb in its natural whole form has many other beneficial properties. For example rose hips is vitamin C in its natural state. Herbs cure disease. Consequently if we eat natural foods (raw as possible) we would rarely get sick. And herbs (plants and food) are packed with usable vitamins and minerals.

Below is a listing of ailments and the corresponding herbs that aid in their treatment. Also where applicable food and food programs will be recommended. For the more serious ailments and illnesses always consult with a knowledgeable herbalist or other health professional.

AILMENT OR HEALTH CONCERN	HERBS & OTHER INFORMATION
Acne/Skin	Chaparral, dandelion, echinacea

Adrenals	Licorice
AIDS	Golden seal, pau d'arco, echinacea, garlic, rose hips, combine with a colon cleanser (e.g. cascara sagrada, senna or psyllium)
Alertness (Staying awake)	Ginseng, ginkgo, gota kola, licorice root, oil of lemon (inhale)
Alcohol Habit (Abuse)	Licorice, dandelion;
Allergies/Sinus	Bayberry, bee pollen; clean blood with yellowdock, burdock or other blood cleanser.
Arteriosclerosis	Garlic, capsicum, hawthorn
Alzheimer's	Gota kola, lecithin, ginkgo
Anemia	Kelp, spirulina, iron supplement; also prunes, sunflower seeds, figs, molasses, and beets all have iron
Appendix Problems	Buckthorn, cascara sagrada
Appetite (Improve)	Alfalfa, camomile, peppermint, fennel
Appetite (Reduce)	Spirulina, chickweed, fennel
Arthritis	Alfalfa, burdock, comfrey, yucca; eat no animal products
Asthma	Mullein and lobelia (taken together), camomile, bayberry, hyssop, comfrey; herba santa
Atherosclerosis	Garlic, cayenne; lecithin
Athlete's Foot	Camomile, safflower; clean colon
Attention Deficit Disorder (ADD)	Catnip, Hops, minerals
Back Sprain	Comfrey and valerian (together) or shavegrass and wild lettuce (together)
Bed Wetting	Cornsilk, uva ursi, peach bark
Bladder Infection	Juniper berries, cornsilk, plantain
Blood Poisoning	Echinacea, chickweed, golden seal
Blood Pressure	Cayenne, garlic, hyssop

Blood Purifiers	Burdock (arthritis); dandelion (liver, addictions, and build the blood); chaparral (skin); echinacea (entire body), garlic, chaparral, red clover
Boils	Echinacea, garlic, golden seal
Bones	Comfrey, horsetail; also eat foods and take supplements rich in vitamin C and the mineral calcium
Brain	Gota kola, blessed thistle, ginkgo
Bronchitis	Comfrey, eucalyptus, lobelia, cayenne
Bruises	Comfrey, cayenne, dandelion, lavender (apply topically)
Burns	Aloe vera; a good salve (topical for healing)
Bursitis	Alfalfa, chaparral, comfrey
Caffeine Addiction	Licorice, dandelion;
Cancer/Tumors	Pau d'arco, golden seal, echinacea; chaparral and red clover combination; don't eat animal products, drink fruit (e.g. lemons) and vegetable (e.g. carrot) juices
Cancer Sore	Myrrh, golden seal
Cataracts	Chaparral, eyebright, gota kola
Chicken Pox	Golden seal, echinacea; NSP: INX or IGS; also eat no animal products
Child Birth (Before)	Red raspberry, squaw vine
Child Birth (After)	Red raspberry
Chronic Fatigue Syndrome	B-Complex, Vitamin A, C, E , garlic
Childhood Diseases	Golden seal, echinacea; yarrow, rosehips and licorice (together)
Cholesterol	Echinacea, hawthorn berries
Circulation	Cayenne, garlic, golden seal
Cleanser (General Body)	Garlic, golden seal
Colds	Peppermint, lemon grass, mullein, bayberry;
Cold Hands or Feet	Cayenne, sage

Colitis	Comfrey, slippery elm;
Colon	Senna, cascara sagrada, aloe vera, or psyllium
Constipation	Burdock, red clover, (mild constipation); psyllium, cascara sagrada, senna, aloe vera (severe constipation)
Cracked Lips	Parsley, garlic, fenugreek
Dandruff	Anise, rosemary, Jojoba oil
Diabetes	Dandelion, golden seal, uva ursi; intelligent eating and exercise
Diarrhea	Psyllium, marshmallow
Digestion	Papaya, peppermint
Digestive Disorders	Safflower, peppermint, ginger, papaya
Diuretic	Juniper berries, parsley, uva ursi
Dizziness	Yellowdock, dandelion, chaparral
Drug Withdrawal	Dandelion, licorice;
Earaches	Lobelia, hops, valerian
Ear Infection	Golden seal; garlic oil (put in ear)
Eczema	Comfrey, burdock, echinacea, chaparral yellowdock
Emphysema	Lobelia, mullein, comfrey (can be taken together); NSP: ALJ (stop smoking)
Energy (Lack of)	Ginseng, bee pollen, ginkgo, royal jelly, gota kola, green additives (barley green, wheat grass, chlorella); clean the colon and the blood; vitamins C and B-complex
Epilepsy	Skullcap, fennel, lobelia
Eye Problems	Bayberry, eyebright
Fasting	Spirulina, licorice; fruit and vegetable juices; food additives (green drinks)
Fever	Peppermint, fresh garlic, rose hips, echinacea
Fibroid Tumors	Red raspberry, don quai; taheebo, chaparral and red clover

Foot Problems	Comfrey foot soak, comfrey and paul d'arco; don't wear tight shoes
Flu	Golden seal, echinacea, peppermint tea and lemon (together)
Fractures	Comfrey, horsetail, slippery elm
Gall Bladder	Golden seal, dandelion, peppermint, buckthorn, comfrey
Gas	Ginger, peppermint, fennel
Glaucoma	Eyebright, alfalfa, fenugreek
Gout	Burdock, safflower
Gray Hair	Horsetail, kelp, oat straw
Gums	Black walnut, comfrey, myrrh
Hair Growth	Horsetail, alfalfa; massage scalp
Hair Health	Alfalfa, sage, kelp, horsetail
Halitosis (Bad breath)	Myrrh, chlorophyll; clean colon
Hangover	Capsicum, wood betony, echinacea, skullcap
Hay fever	Bee pollen, cayenne, alfalfa
Headache	Camomile, valerian, fenugreek and thyme (together)
Heat (Excess body)	Aloe vera, mint herbs (spearmint or peppermint)
Heart	Garlic, cayenne pepper, hawthorn; clean blood
Heartburn	Peppermint, sasparilla, papaya, fennel
Hemorrhage(Internal or External	Cayenne, golden seal
Hemorrhoids	Uva ursi, shepherd's purse
Hepatitis	White oak bark, dandelion, cayenne
Hernia	Red clover, chaparral, clean colon with herbs (aloe vera, senna, etc.)
Herpes	Golden seal, black walnut, myrrh;
High Blood Pressure	Garlic, cayenne, ginseng, golden seal
Hoarseness	Bayberry, mullein, licorice
Hormone (Female)	Dong quai, damiana, blue cohosh, black cohosh

Hormone (Male)	Ginseng, saw palmetto;
Hyperactivity	Valerian, hops, skullcap; if children are hyperactive stop feeding them sugar
Hypoglycemia	Dandelion, licorice, safflower
Immune System	Golden seal, fresh garlic, echinacea, vitamins A, E, and C (rose hips);
Impotence	Ginseng, licorice;
Infection	Echinacea, golden seal
Infertility	Red raspberry, blue cohosh (together);
Inflammation	Echinacea, comfrey, slippery elm
Insect bites	Echinacea, black cohosh
Insomnia	Camomile, skullcap, catnip, valerian,
Insulin	Golden seal (it stimulates the pancreas to produce insulin)
Intestines	Acidophilus
Itching	Yellowdock, plantain, herbal oil
Jaundice	Dandelion, wood betony
Kidneys/Urinary tract	Marshmallow root, juniper berries, uva ursi; watermelon or cranberry juice
Lactation (Decrease	Parsley, sage
Lactation (increase)	Blessed thistle, marshmallow
Lime Disease	Vitamin A, E, C, Evening Primrose oil, Garlic
Liver	Barberry, Dandelion, Vitamin D
Longevity	Ginseng, ginkgo, gota kola
Low Blood Pressure	Cayenne, dandelion, garlic
Lungs	Mullein and lobelia (together), comfrey, fenugreek; NSP: LH or herba santa
Lupus	Dandelion, yellowdock, red clover
Lymphatic System	Echinacea, yellowdock; chaparral and red clover (together); eat less animal products
Memory	Ginkgo, gota kola

Menopause	Black cohosh, false unicorn, blessed thistle
Menstrual Cramps	Red raspberry, camomile, peppermint;
Menstrual Problems	Red raspberry;
Mental fatigue	Ginkgo, ginseng
Migraine Headaches	Camomile, lobelia
Morning Sickness	Ginger root, peppermint
Motion Sickness	Peppermint, skullcap, catnip, valerian
Mouth Problems	Aloe vera, golden seal
Mucous	Bayberry, mullein, golden seal, echinacea; eat less animal products
Muscle Cramps	Comfrey, dandelion, alfalfa
Muscular Dystrophy	B-Complex vitamin, Kelp
Muscle Spasms	Oat straw, lobelia, catnip
Multiple Sclerosis	Lobelia, hops, valerian
Nails	Horsetail;
Nausea	Catnip, peppermint
Nervous Disorders	Skullcap, catnip, hops, valerian; reduce sugar intake; C and B vitamins
Nightmares	Skullcap, hops
Nose Congestion	Peppermint, spearmint, eucalyptus
Odors (Body)	Chlorophyll
Pain	Camomile, valerian, wild lettuce; comfrey and mullein (together);
Pancreas	Golden seal, uva ursi;
Parasites	Black walnut, herbal pumpkin, fresh garlic; pumpkin seeds
Poison Ivy	Mullein, yellow dock
Perspiration (Promote)	Ginger, hyssop, sage
Pregnancy (during)	Red raspberry;
Prostrate Problems	Golden Seal, pumpkin seeds, ginger;
Psoriasis	Burdock, chaparral, dandelion, sasparilla; clean colon
Relaxers	Camomile, hops, valerian, skullcap
Rheumatism	Burdock, alfalfa

Ringworm	Black walnut, golden seal
Sarcoidosis	Mullein and lobelia (together); echinacea and passion flower (together); also clean colon
Senility	Gota kola, ginseng, ginkgo
Senses (Enhance)	Ginseng, kelp, any nervine herbs (e.g. hops, skullcap)
Sexual Depressant	Skullcap, hops; keep colon clean; eat lots of green vegetables (mostly raw); eat no animal products
Sexual Stimulant	Ginseng, saw palmetto, damiana (together)
Sexually Transmitted Diseases	Golden seal, echinacea, red clover (all can be taken together); also change the diet to quality foods
Shock	Cayenne, lobelia
Sickle Cell Anemia	Dandelion (liver and blood), aloe vera or senna (colon cleanser), and chaparral or echinacea (blood purifier) (together)
Skin (Dry)	Chickweed, dandelion, horsetail, camomile, yellowdock, chaparral, red clover, and olive oil can be used externally and internally; also evening primrose oil and wheat germ oil as well as vitamins A and E are good for the skin
Skin (Oily)	Horsetail, burdock, aloe vera, dandelion, golden seal, red clover; vitamins A and E are good for the skin
Smoking Habit	Catnip, skullcap, peppermint
Spasms	Catnip, blue cohosh, lobelia
Spinal Meningitis	Golden seal, lobelia
Spleen	Dandelion, golden seal
Stomach Cramps	Camomile, peppermint, slippery elm
Stomach Problems	Papaya, peppermint;

Stress	Skullcap, camomile, hops, valerian; NSP: Nutricalm; vitamins C and B-complex
Sugar Habit	Dandelion, licorice; CCI: Correction Connection
Teeth	Comfrey, black walnut
Throat Soreness or Irritation	Golden seal, cayenne, garlic; licorice extract
Tonsillitis	Echinacea, golden seal
Toothache	Cloves, lobelia, mullein and comfrey (together)
Thyroid	Kelp, irish moss
Ulcers	Cayenne, golden seal, myrrh
Uplift Spirits	Ginseng, blue cohosh; oil of rose, rosemary, or lavender (inhale or apply topically)
Uterus/Ovaries	False unicorn, red raspberry, don quai
Vaginal Douche	Marshmallow, slippery elm, uva ursi
Vaginal Infection	Red raspberry, golden seal;
Vaginal Soreness	Aloe vera gel (applied topically)
Wart	Mullein, chaparral
Water Retention	Uva ursi, cornsilk, parsley
Weight Gain	Camomile, alfalfa, ginseng, golden seal;
Weight Loss	Spirulina, chickweed, and cascara sagrada (together)
Yeast Infection	Acidophilus; NSP :eat no animal products

The herbs recommended work best when one begins to change their diet to wholesome foods. If you are sick or have been recommended to have an operation, try the herbs first. Seek the advice of someone who is very familiar with herbs and other alternative therapies. The herbs may take several weeks to do their work, but they do work. However, sometimes one may have to try more than one herb to get the desired results.

It is not our intent to openly prescribe or give medical advice. We have recommended that you seek the advice of more than one health professional (herbalist, doctor, chiropractor, etc.). If you utilize this information with or without your doctor's or other health advisor's knowledge, you are treating yourself which is your right and choice.

Organically Grown Foods

We must understand the necessity of having a pure body and an earth free of deadly chemicals and drugs. Foods that are sprayed with pesticides damage the body and deplete the immune system. These chemicals are disease causing agents which stay in the body, accelerating the aging process.

Many food growers spray fruit trees with chemicals to accelerate their growth. Plants are grown in chemicalized soil and fertilizer. They also wax or spray fruits and vegetables with chemicals that preserve or maintain color (e.g. alar in apples). Animals are fed chemicalized food and are themselves injected with drugs to make them grow faster and bigger, reproduce better, and have leaner meat.

Spraying chemicals and pesticides on crops will only work in the short term because insects can buildup a resistance to many drugs. Although the crop yields from chemicalized farming may initially be greater, eventually the soil becomes depleted and its future usefulness is minimized.

Organic farming replenishes the earth. The soil is fertilized with natural manure. The insects are controlled through natural means. Organic foods are not sprayed or processed after they are picked. Organic fruits and vegetables are free of all chemicals and are grown with the highest ecological standards. Organic farming allows the body to get the maximum benefit of the food.

Many farmers are slowly turning to organic foods. Organic methods of farming are cheaper in the long term. Organic farming helps maintain the soil and extends its useful life. Ultimately more people can be fed and the earth preserved with organic farming.

Organic foods taste better and fresher. Most health food stores as well as fruit and vegetable outlets are familiar with the farmers. They are aware of how they grow their food and maintain the soil. Organic foods may cost a little more but the value of good health is priceless.

Raw Foods

When most people think of raw foods they probably envision eating raw meat or eating foods that couldn't possibly taste good. Both are untrue. Raw foods are foods eaten in their natural state (uncooked).

First, if you eat meat it would be wise to cook it. Secondly taste buds are trained to choose different foods but they can be retrained. It is very wise to consider this since the more raw foods that we eat, the healthier we will be.

Man up to a few hundreds years ago ate almost all raw foods and very little animal flesh. However, all animals eat their food raw. Even carnivores animals who are the only species of life who are anatomically designed to eat flesh (they have the teeth and digestive system to properly handle it while humans don't) eat their food raw. Additionally, humans can more easily chew and digest fowl and fish (baked, broiled or fried in high quality cooking oil) much easier than other flesh.

It normally takes eight hours to digest fowl and fish while other flesh takes up to seventy two hours to digest. But the raw foods which humans should consume are fruits, nuts, legumes and vegetables. Raw foods have maximum nutrition. We eat to nutrify the body. Raw food contains vitamins, minerals, and protein that the body needs to enliven itself, protect us from diseases and grow.

When we cook the food we minimize its nutritional benefit to the body. We actually can destroy these nutrients (by cooking) to the extent that the food has almost no value to the body and when ingested represents mostly waste matter that the body must struggle to get rid of. So cook only fresh vegetables, grain, and flesh (chicken, turkey, and fish).

Eat a raw vegetable salad at every meal. And eat as much fruit as possible. Keep your cooked vegetables in their natural juices and you can drink the juice. That's where most of the nutrition ends up after cooking. Also grains (rice, bread, etc.) must be cooked. They have a good amount of calcium, B-complex vitamins and other nutrients.

Raw foods and salads should make up thirty to forty percent of our daily food intake. That's just a middle of the road goal. The more raw food that we eat the faster we tend to eliminate our waste. Consequently, the blood and the body are not polluted. We get the full nutritional benefit and, of course, we feel good.

In the recipe section of this book there are several completely raw and semi-raw dishes in the Raw Food and Salads section. Try as many as you desire.

Positive Food Additives

A properly nutrified body is strong enough to withstand stress, defeat addiction, control weight and to maintain good overall health. There are certain foods, herbs,and formulas which help restore health, rebuild the body, and cure ailments. These additives also provide valuable nutrients that our diet may not supply.

The Correction Connection products, Bahamian Diet (for weight loss) and the Correction Connection formula (for habits and addictions) are very good vitamin and mineral supplements with a soya (protein) base. Nature's Sunshine has many effective herbal, vitamin, and mineral supplement formulas. It also has quality single herbs that can help specific body organs. Nature's Plus, Nature's Way, and Nature's Herbs products have good supplements and herbal blends.

The Sunrider, Omni IV and Km products have good nutrition and herbal supplements. When choosing supplements read labels to find out the ingredients in each product. A good supplement contains no fillers, artificial colors or flavors or any other potentially health-debilitating ingredients. There are many other companies that offer effective formulas for various ailments. The local health food store and wholistic health professionals are great resources and have a wealth of information on various food additives and health issues.

Chlorella, barleygreen and wheatgrass are green foods that excellently enhance the body. These foods have been known to enhance the immune system, clean the blood, regulate weight and to provide all the nutrients that the body needs, (chlorophyll, protein, vitamins, minerals and other nutrients). Chlorophyll helps the body in the healing of wounds and burns, tones the stomach and helps eliminate harmful chemicals and metals in the body. It tends to increase the red blood cell count and eliminates body odors.

Some other great additives are the products of the bee, namely, bee pollen, royal jelly, and propolis. These products are a source of body energy and enhancement. They are rich in all nutrients (vitamins, minerals, and proteins). They have been used to cure many ailments including diabetes, heart problems and allergies.

Lecithin is a very good additive. It is important in the function of the nerves, brain, heart, kidneys, and liver. Lecithin is found in every cell in the body, but primarily in the previously mentioned organs. Lecithin may help prevent age-related memory loss. It prevents cholesterol and other fats from accumulating on the walls of the arteries. The best source of lecithin is soya lecithin found in health food stores. Lecithin supplements can make you more youthful and healthier.

One of the most powerful and effective herbs for those who are trying to change their diet or those in transition is echinacea. Echinacea was widely used by the American Indians, herbalists, and early doctors. It is used in Europe and is gaining popularity in America. It is a great blood purifier. It lowers the blood acid level and detoxifies the system (by cleansing the blood and the lymphatic system). It can aid in curing cancer, arthritis, skin problems, and infections. It contains vitamins A, E, and C. (See Illustration of Herb Echinacea on page 126.)

Echinacea can be used for young children and adults. It can be used as an antibiotic and can be used to cure sexually transmitted diseases. It can be used to treat boils, fibroid tumors, and a host of health problems including swellings, growths, sinuses, colds, and the flu.

Golden seal has been successfully used in curing many of the above health problems. It is a blood, body, and organ cleanser especially good for diabetes, colds, liver, kidneys, infections, blood disorders, male genitals, and sexually transmitted diseases.

Garlic is another good blood cleanser which strengthens the heart and the immune system. It also lowers blood pressure. Additionally, it is very good for infections, colds, mucous and a sore throat. Garlic stimulates the appetite, enhances digestion and helps eliminate parasites and germs from the body.

Spirulina is an excellent additive to the diet especially for those trying to lose weight. It contains all of the eight essential amino acids of protein in a very digestive form. It has all B-complex vitamins and is one of the highest known sources of vitamin B-12 (important for vegetarians).

It has a high amount of beta carotene (provitamin A) and iron as well as having all the necessary minerals. It curbs the appetite, reduces sugar cravings, and provides a boost of physical and mental energy while maintaining a balanced blood sugar level. It minimizes hunger during fasting and it is a powerful body cleanser and detoxifier.

Camomile is a preferred herb in tea form along with peppermint. Both clean and strengthen the entire body. Both are very good for colds. Peppermint helps eliminate headache, heartburn, morning sickness, liver problems and promotes the appetite. It is a good digestive aid and also strengthens the bowels.

Peppermint and camomile are pain relievers that are good for menstrual cramps. Both have a soothing affect on the stomach and the entire system. They are very good for the nerves and nervous conditions. Camomile helps relieve tension and overall anxiety. It is a soothing sedative which helps most stomach troubles. It is good for the kidneys and promotes the appetite. It can be used externally to treat bruises, sprains, swellings and open wounds. Peppermint contains calcium, potassium, and magnesium. Camomile has a good amount of calcium and potassium.

Cayenne pepper deserves special mention. It is a powerful blood builder which regulates the blood pressure, cleans the artery walls and strengthens the heart. It is also good for cuts, hemorrhages, wounds, fractures, hemorrhoids, ulcers and all problems related to colds, sore throat and mucous. It can be used internally and externally. For instance, it can be placed in your shoes or gloves during winter months to add warmth.

Cayenne pepper is known by many other names such as red pepper, capsicum, red peppers, Spanish pepper, African pepper, chili pepper, and American red pepper. It is an excellent stimulant that cause no bad health reaction (except it's a little hot). It helps other herbs work better since it enhances blood circulation and all herbs use the blood to travel throughout the body. Cayenne contains vitamins A, C, the minerals calcium, iron, magnesium phorus and sulfur.

Alfalfa is an excellent herb. It is rich in minerals like calcium, phosphorous, iron, and potassium. It is also rich in the trace minerals like chlorine, fluorine, and magnesium, and is a good source of vitamins A, C, D, K and most of the B-complex vitamins. It is a good vitamin and mineral supplement and is effectively used for many areas of the body where the previously mentioned nutrients are critical such as hair, teeth, brain, uterus, pancreas and the digestive system. It is one of the herbs whose roots reach deep into the earth to collect vital nutrients.

Alfalfa is also good for urinary tract and kidney problems. It is good for bowel and intestinal problems. It is a good protein source containing all eight essential amino acids. It is also good for people with alcohol and drug problems.

Dandelion is an excellent herb for blood purification and enhancement. It filters toxins out of the blood stream. It is especially valuable for liver disorders and diabetes. Dandelion is a powerful liver cleanser and also enhances the proper functioning of the spleen, pancreas, and the gall bladder. It can aid in alleviating skin disorders of all kinds. It grows wild in many parks, lawns, and even in your backyard. But most of us wouldn't know what it is.

Dandelion is very nutritious. It is a very good source of protein. It is a good source of vitamins A, C, E, and B_1, B_2, B_3, and the minerals potassium, sodium, calcium, phosphorus, magnesium, iron, and chlorine.

Certain fruits and vegetable juices promote health. We will only discuss carrot juice and lemon juice because they are the most important. Lemons are powerful body cleansers. They help to remove impurities and toxins out of the system. Lemons contain high amounts of vitamin C, calcium and potassium. They are great for colds, flu, sore throat, fever, asthma, liver problems, bones and teeth. They are also good for heartburn, gas, the digestive system and the skin. They will remove most skin discolorations.

Carrot juice is an excellent additive to the diet. It is very pleasant tasting. It promotes healthiness in our entire body, but is especially healing to the lungs, eyes, teeth, digestive and nervous system. It tends to increase and enhance the quality of mother's milk. It contains virtually all of the vitamins (A, B, C, D, E and K), many of the essential amino acids and a significant amount of calcium. It also contains beta carotene, potassium and iron in significant amounts. It is especially good for colds, flu and related health problems. It is a good nutritional supplement. A glass or two a day is sufficient to give you most of your daily nutrition requirements and enhance your body.

Carrot juice can be combined with other vegetable juices to aid in healing certain ailments. The juice of beets (for blood and anemia) celery (for kidneys, liver and arthritis (joints)) and cucumbers (for skin, diuretic and natural insulin) can be combined with carrot juice to make a tasty and healthy beverage.

Proper Rest and Exercise

Our minds and our spirit-selves are challenged regularly with life's difficulties. This makes them stronger and more resilient. Our bodies need challenges and intelligent exercise is a very efficient and effective means for most of us to give the body what it needs.

Proper exercise is very important for good health. It tends to strengthen the heart. It helps the blood to cleanse itself and do its job better. It tends to remove toxins and waste from the body because we sweat (eliminate waste). Consequently, we have more energy.

Exercise also enhances muscles and tissue development. It helps all eliminative organs (lungs, kidneys, skin, and the colon) to clear the waste out of the body. Hence the organs work more efficiently. Recent studies have shown that regular exercise improves health.

Anyone can exercise from the very young to the very old. Different exercises work better or may be safer for different people. Check with your health advisor for the proper exercises for you.

Some of the less strenuous exercises include walking, stationery bike riding, stretching, and light calisthenics. Aerobics classes include exercises for most body parts and are an excellent means of staying in shape. More strenuous exercises such as weight lifting, jogging, outdoor bike riding, and swimming are great for the body.

Exercise plays a great role in weight loss programs. It helps burn fat and enhances the activities of the digestive organs. Hence one tends to eliminate better.

Athletes and those who moderately exercise need more vitamins, minerals, and aminos (proteins) than the average person. The sweating, muscle work and general activity takes nutrients out of the body.

Specific minerals like calcium, magnesium, zinc, potassium, and chromium and the water soluble vitamins C and B-complex are easily leeched out of the body during exercise. It is very difficult to get these nutrients in the amounts needed through the foods that we eat so natural supplements are a must.

Athletes and exercisers should take a sufficient amount of provitamin A (beta carotene), B-complex, C and E. The amounts required for each person may vary so one may want to take a little more than the recommended daily allowance.

The best and most convenient way to get the adequate amount of nutrients is to take certain herbs and a good multivitamin and mineral supplement. Herbs like alfalfa, rose hips, kelp, and spirulina are packed with vitamins and minerals.

Ginseng, bee pollen, and/or royal jelly provide needed energy for exercise and also have most of the necessary nutrients.

There are many vitamin, herb, and whole food companies that sell good multivitamin and mineral supplements.

Exercise also plays a significant role in helping the body overcome the stress of broken bones and damaged tissue by strengthening them. It also helps the body defeat certain health maladies such as colds, heart problems, arthritis, and diabetes. Exercise also helps us to look and feel younger. Ironically the more improper foods that one eats, the less motivation and energy one will have to exercise.

Proper rest is a critical component of good health. The body needs quiet time, too. Rest allows tissue muscles and organs to relax and rebuild themselves. The body can draw upon the inner force's divine energies. The Creator's divine sunlight can shine on our spiritual selves.

Inspiration can enliven our conscious minds with answers to problems and reaffirmations for strength. Rest relaxes the body and mind after the day's stress and challenges. This allows the body to renew and refresh itself without the worlds demands on us and or time.

Although we have been told that we need 8 hours of sleep our bodies can survive in good health with only 4-6 hours of sleep. The diet has a lot to do with our sleep requirements. A healthy body with a rather clean colon and circulation system needs much less than 8 hours.

Fasting and Massage

Massage is an excellent therapeutic tool for the body. It relaxes muscles and releases tensions. It reduces stress and anxiety. It produces a peaceful state in the body.

There are many different types of massage therapies. There is the shiatsu massage, swedish massage, and other methods. There are massages for health, stress reduction, sensuality, and spiritual enhancement. Massages can be utilized to relax muscles, to aid in healing, and to strengthen bones and limbs.

Many professional massage therapists exist in every part of America. Many chiropractors use massage techniques as well as making spinal and back adjustments. Naprapaths use massage, supplements, and nutrition to bring about wellness.

Foot massage is a very popular means of relaxation and stress reduction. The foot is one of the nerve ending points where the health status can be evaluated. There is power in touching. And we can release negative energy through touching. And we can heal through touching, rubbing, and manipulating parts of the body.

Fasting is another key component of a healthy lifestyle. Fasting is denying yourself food and/or liquids for a period of time. The three main reasons for fasting are cleansing (physical, mental, and spiritual), discipline, and to eliminate illness.

Fasting allows the body to heal itself without being disturbed. It gives the body a chance to rest and be peaceful. It allows the God force within our bodies to manifest and give us right guidance and inspiration. Also our minds are keen and aware during fasts.

There are basically three popular fasts. A fruit fast is an easy and a most popular fast. It consists of eating fruits both subacid (prunes, dates, bananas, apples, cherries, grapes, peaches, plums, etc.) and alkaline (honeydew, cantaloupe, watermelon) and drinking pure water and juice (both fruit and vegetable). Also, lemons, oranges and grape fruit are acidic fruits which are nutritiously useful during a fast. There is a liquid fast where only liquids are consumed. Then there is a type of fast where one consumes nothing but maybe a little water.

Fasting can help you lose weight, heal your body, and gain more self control. There is a spiritual awakening or enhancement that takes place when one fasts. All scripture mention fasting as a means of getting closer to the Creator and the inner self. We need to be in contact with our innerselves, since our normal daily activities act as a distraction to our acquaintance with this vital part of our existence.

Fasting helps us create a healthy and positive frame of mind. It gives us the freedom to refocus and concentrate on the more important realities of life. One should consult their health advisor or do research for the best fasting program.

The Way Back

They ask thee what is lawful to them as food. Say: lawful to you are all things good and pure. Quran 5:4

Innerviews

The body is a perfect machine. It is the physical manifestation of the Great Perfect Intelligence that created everything in the universe. The Creative Force whether you call Him Yahweh, Almighty God, Jehovah, Allah, the Universal Force or whatever, wants the best for man. We should want the best for ourselves.

The earth is a divine test for man. So far we've been largely failing the test. We have plundered the earth and abused ourselves with the thoughts only of pleasure and profit on the material plane. The result is what we see today.

The violence, drug addictions, hatred, jealousy, confusion, resentment, stress and wars are directly the results of the violation of our bodies and the earth. When you consume bad food you pollute the body, the mind, and the spirit. And within ourselves we must each make changes to bring about the wholesomeness that we all want.

For if we eat more wholesome food we will be more whole, complete, fulfilled, and energized. Just like there are laws in the universe, there are laws that govern the body. Proper diet is the foundation. Proper rest and exercise are important. Then we need a positive mental attitude and a fairly stable environment. Not a perfect one.

Perfection should be our goal both within ourselves and in the environment. It does take effort. But the rewards make it worth the while.

We should realize that perfection is largely the result of struggle against adversity. We can conceive of perfection outside ourselves. We wear the perfect looking outfit and want to drive the perfect car. We revere perfect sports heroes whether they are Julius Erving, Michael Jordan, or Wayne Gretsky. We are in awe at the technological advancements such as the computer.

We can visualize perfection outside of ourselves but what about within?

Man is the creator of perfection outside of himself and also within. The outward is just an example of the perfect potential within. Inward development enhances the outer possibilities. But there are laws that must be followed in evolving spiritually or physically.

The laws governing the body are basic and easy to follow for the most part. The problem is that most people have bad habits which are hard to break. Eating too many denatured, processed foods high in sugar, salt, fats, and drugs is what must be changed. It's not easy but it's not that difficult. I know because I have overcome most of my bad habits and I'm still working on some. And it's a process of continuing to struggle for complete self control. All habits can be changed. The first step is to make a conscious decision and then start down the road. There are supportive factors that will aid in your making changes. You just need to have faith and keep moving in the right direction.

Your health is your responsibility unless you are a child. In any case you will suffer the consequences of your actions. Neither the doctor or anyone else can feel your discomfort or pain. You have the opportunity to achieve optimal health.

We must reprogram our minds and renourish our spirits. We must communicate with positive people and perform as many giving acts as possible. Giving enhances the possibilities for healing. We must make a commitment to having harmony in our lives. Sometimes in order to get to harmony we must go through some conflict. But peace and harmony must be our vision and our goal. Each day's successes or failures should not deter us from the goals that we have set.

Most of us need motivation and encouragement in making these transitions. A supporting environment is a great foundation for change. But if one does not have the best environment change just takes more effort.

One should strive to create an aura of positiveness and peace around them. This comes through prayer, meditation, visualization, and contagioning your environment with positive affirmations. The mind is so powerful that it can possibly produce the image that one dwells upon in reality. This belief system is not new. We heard the saying "as a man thinks so is he." Father Divine repeatedly said what one visualizes can be materialized. And Christ, the most renown positive imager of all said when he healed "by your faith you are healed" meaning that the sick person must believe themselves well.

Remember, disease and ill-health have a mental and physical component. A proper diet will help us withstand any mental trauma. And it enhances the possibilities for spiritual development.

No one gives anyone bad health although one can be the igniter of bad health in another. In other words, if you get a cold, flu, venereal disease, or any other so-called contagious disease, the seed bed for that disease is within you. Communicable disease is a communicating of dis-ease between two active participants, both physically and spiritually.

Health Tips for the Wise

The following are 32 pertinent health-related suggestions. They can be used as a quick reference for those who want more information. The wise are those who want to make changes in their diet and need more information.

1. Whatever you do stop eating white refined sugar. It is a drug and a poison. It causes many of the health maladies that we experience. Pure, unprocessed honey, raw sugar, barley malt, pure maple syrup, rice syrup, and molasses are more viable options.

2. Eliminate pork and beef in the diet. They contain uric acid (urine) from the animal and are injected with many drugs. Pork is scripturally prohibited and beef should be forbidden also. They both cause heart and blood problems and may impair the proper functioning of all organs. They cause cancer and other diseases of the spirit and the body.

3. Chicken and turkey are good in transition. They too are injected with some drugs. They along with fish (boned or scaled) are a very viable alternative to pork and beef. Turkey has one-third less fat than chicken. Eat kosher or halal chicken or turkey.

4) Dairy products are toxic to the system. They fill the body up with mucous. Dairy products are the cause of various ailments directly or indirectly (mumps, measles, chicken pox, flu, sinus difficulties, lung, heart, thyroid, colds, uterus, and genital problems).

5. Feed your children very few animal products if you want them to be healthy. Many products that adults and children eat are laden with sugar, chemicals, and other questionable ingredients (artificial colorings and flavorings). Breast-feed your babies as long as possible.

6. Read labels. Ask questions about foods. Read periodicals. Watch the disguised ingredients in foods (e.g. sugar called invert sugar, high fructose syrup, corn syrup, brown sugar, etc.).

7. Salt and other seasonings in excess are unhealthy. They interfere with digestion, damage the heart, cause cancer, and pollute the blood. Use sea salt and natural seasonings (in moderation).

8. Bake, broil, boil, or stew fish, chicken, or turkey. If you do fry food, fry in quality oils such as safflower, sunflower, sesame, corn, or olive oil. Avoid all barbecued food.

9. Eat as much fresh and raw (uncooked) fruits, vegetables, nuts, seeds, etc. as possible. Cooking minimizes the nutritional benefits of foods. So lightly cook or steam vegetables if you must cook them.

10. Eat raw vegetable salads at least once a day. Some great veggies to put in salads are lettuce (romaine), cabbage, carrots, scallions, onions, cucumbers, radishes, sprouts, and tomatoes. Those veggies are very nutritious. Iceberg lettuce has little nutritional value but is not a harmful food.

11. Oils are very valuable to the system. They lubricate the system and provide nutrition. They are a good source of vegetable fats and vitamin E. Most oils aid digestion and lubricate the bowels. Most salad dressings (vegetarian) have oils in them. Use in moderation.

12. Combine foods intelligently. Eat raw vegetables first, then cooked vegetables, then grains and protein can be eaten together. Don't eat fruit with other foods. Wait an hour between eating fruits and other foods.

13. Don't eat and drink at the same time. You'll confuse your digestive system and won't get the full benefits of your food. Wait one half hour to an hour between eating and drinking. Drink 6-8 glasses of water daily.

14. Eat slowly. Eat for nutrition as well as to fill your stomach. Pray or meditate over food. Chew your food properly (e.g. 20-30 times).

15. Don't eat while under stress. Calm yourself down before you eat. Proper foods enhance your ability to defeat stress.

16. Drink tap water only through a good water filter (e.g. C.C.I.'s water filtration system). Spring water is a better alternative provided that it comes from a pure source.

17. Take herbal formulas, vitamin and mineral supplements, and/or food additives. The following are examples: garlic, wheat grass, cholerella, rose hips, barley green, ginseng, bee pollen, and royal jelly. Vitamin and mineral deficiencies are the cause of many diseases and addictions.

18. Keep the colon moving. Take the colon cleansing herbs (e.g. senna, psyllium, aloe vera, cascara sagrada). Acidophilus replaces the friendly bacteria if you get high enemas or colonics. A healthy colon is the first step in good health.

19.   Take extra water soluble vitamins B-complex and C especially if under stress. Also make sure you are getting enough quality foods that have non dairy calcium (e.g. soya products, grains and most vegetables).

20.   Massage may be important to good health. It invigorates the body and the mind. Try to get one regularly. Most aromatic herbs are very good in massage therapy.

21.   Don't eat out of aluminum pots, pans, and other utensils. Eating foods out of aluminum containers may eventually cause alzheimer's disease, cancer, and other ailments. Use cast iron or stainless steel cooking utensils. Don't eat irradiated foods.

22.   Know your own body. Gradual changes are better than quick changes. But always change for the better.

23.   Try not to eat after 9:00 PM except fruit and easily digested foods; don't eat anything but fruits before 11:00 AM. Remember it's not what you do every once in a while but what you do regularly that causes the real damage.

24.   There are good food substitutes for every bad food that we eat. The health food stores and magazines can provide you with much of the good food information.

25.   Don't overeat. We can live on one main meal and one or two smaller meals. Don't eat too much protein especially animal products. Eat very few canned foods and few condiments (ketchup, relish, mustard, etc.).

26.   If you have carefully read this book I am suggesting similar foods and herbs to get well and stay well with few exceptions. Most diseases have a similar origin, namely, a polluted bloodstream and an impacted colon. These conditions affect the entire body from head to foot.

27.   When you first clean the waste out of your body with herbs and if you are very toxic (full of waste), you might experience an adverse cleansing reaction (e.g. nausea, low energy, or headaches). Don't panic. Cleansing reactions affect a small number of people and usually last a couple of days. When it's over you'll be a better and healthier person. Always check with your health advisor to make sure that you are not doing anything wrong.

28.   Most doctors don't know about herbs and don't recommend them. There are many health professionals (including some doctors) who have knowledge of nutrition and herbs. Consult with them.

29.   A good image and appearance are important in the business world. Eating quality foods, taking food additives, and

exercising maintains youthfulness and enhancing appearance so corporations should have an interest in the dietary habits of their employees. Also less people would take a sick day for illnesses (increasing profits and productivity). And people would be more mentally alert and less tired making them more productive.

30.   Remember the good, better and best principle. Good is making the critical changes in your diet and moving toward the better. Better is arriving at a point where you eat only high quality foods in the best manner possible. The best is when you have almost complete discipline and you are knowledgeable of all aspects of food, diet, and related activities. You fast regularly and are aware of your inner nature.

31.   The body is self-healing. It just needs the proper environment (inner and outer) to grow. Make the right moves and you will be blessed with success. Strive hard and get the best out of life and the best will come back.

32.   Belief in positive thinking and practicing strong meditative affirmations are powerful in defeating health problems and any other problems. Subliminal tapes (e.g. ocean waves) and constantly repeating positive affirmations are powerful tools for having a good outlook of life.

Some Wholistic Approaches

The wholistic approach to health care means treating the total person (mind, body and spirit). Almost all diseases have a spiritual cause though their effects may be based or centered in the physical body. If a health practitioner treats the entire person, they will be much more effective in establishing and maintaining a total state of well-being in their patients. Counseling, prayer, meditation, and positive affirmations are ways of resolving mental, emotional, and spiritual conflicts.

The following is a list of methods and disciplines that aid in producing wellness for the total person. They represent approaches to and tools for healing. By no means is this a complete list. But it includes the more viable and effective tools for healing.

1. *Acupuncture-* It is a Chinese healing system that seeks to balance the energy flow within the body using needles and heat treatments. It has been used to alleviate pain, headaches, and many other ailments.

2. *Chiropractic-* The alignment of the body by using techniques which involve the spine and the careful adjustment of the spine. Also it includes the careful adjustment of bones to heal

fractures and bruises. Today some chiropractors use massage therapy as an additional tool in promoting wellness.

3. *Homeopathy-* A system of treatment of illnesses that is centered in the belief that like cures like. Homeopathic doctors use medicines which are strongly herbally based. In fact a homeopathic doctor utilizes traditional medical approaches and herbal (and wholistic) approaches.

4. *Iridology -* A means of diagnosing conditions in the individual by examining the iris of the eye, then herb and food programs can be recommended.

5. *Naprapathy-* A system of gentle manipulations and specific stretching of all joints and the spine to restore mobility in the tissue.

6. *Naturopathy-* Using natural means to assist in healing. Some of the traditional medicinal diagnostic methods such as herbal remedies may be used. However, treatments only consist of wholistic methods.

7. *Herbology-* Treating illnesses and healing the body with herbs.

School of Common Sense

This section is written to emphasize and verify that there is a common sense logical approach to health. There is nothing complicated about health and the human body. We just need to do a little research to know how to maintain our bodies.

Let's go through a series of logical questions which hopefully will allow you to see that we all play a part in the plan to bring about wellness.

1. If this body that we say is ours is priceless then why do we violate it consistently with bad food, drugs, and improper maintenance?

2. Why is it that 100 years ago incidence of cancer, diabetes, sinus difficulties, and heart problems were rare and today with all the technological, sophisticated medical advances these health problems are replete in the nation?

3. Why do we want the best quality clothes, car, house, appearance, mate, etc. then we short change ourselves when it comes to our diet?

4. Why is it that Hippocrates, who is the father of western medicine, was a naturopathic doctor.

5. If meat is a better protein and humans need so much of it why do most of the biggest and strongest animals (elephant, hippo, rhino, horse, etc.) practice vegetarianism and don't need animal products to survive?

6.   If the Bible says that it is a sin to violate your body temple with alcohol and illegal drugs (cocaine, etc.) what about legal drugs such as coffee, sugar, tobacco, and pharmaceuticals (aspirin, etc.)? Does your body know the difference?

7.   Doesn't the natural in natural food imply that these are foods we should be eating?

8.   If cancer (and AIDS) attack and deplete the immune system,then if there are foods, herbs, and vitamins that strengthen the immune system shouldn't we be taking these substances?

9.   Does the Creator desire wellness or sickness for us?

10. If you believe that what I am saying is true then why not start now to improve your life?

By no means is this book attacking the medical industry. Many of the services and functions that this industry performs are valuable and necessary. But many are very questionable and in some cases dangerous. The medical industry rejects the great majority of natural approaches to health care. They label them unproven, ineffective, and unnecessary, but the natural methods are thousands of years old whereas modern medicine is a few hundred years old. Modern medicine seems to be more concerned with controlling sickness after it ensues. The natural methods emphasize disease prevention and quick action to eliminate it if it occurs. With so many sick people in America, there must be something wrong.

We are coming into a new age. An age where all the blinders can be taken off your eyes if that is what you desire. An age where some of the traditional laws must be put back in action. The information is available to us to know what to do.

It is very ironic that the Chinese and Japanese in particular and most oriental people in general have a more balanced and nutritious diet than Americans. Japan and China can boast of having some of the world's oldest people. Eating is not approached with the same passionate fervor in China. The Chinese people eat more whole grains, vegetables, fruit, and simple food. They have a very structured, systematic, effective way of producing food. In fact China the world's largest nation, imports very little food although it is a poor country.

The Japanese diet is similar although Japan is one of the world's great economic powers. The Japanese eat a lot of sea vegetables such as kombu, sushi, arrame, etc. They eat a lot of fish instead of beef and pork. The Japanese and Chinese eat a lot of rice and are familiar with and/or take herbs.

Both peoples tend to respect the needs of the inner person as well as the outer person. Both peoples tend to respect the earth and are more in harmony with it than us. Does that explain their healthier lifestyle where sickness is not as prevalent as here? And we are well aware of the industriousness of these peoples. They emphasize production, cooperation, industry, and success in their culture, not despair, disharmony, greed, unintelligent freedoms and sickness. They are more successful and we materially have more. Isn't that ironical?

Can't we do better as a nation?

The information contained in this writing is very valuable. But I don't expect everyone to accept what I say at face value. There are plenty of reference sources in the back of this book. This leaves the challenge up to you. Make the changes that you can. Do some reading. And don't forget the best.

My desire is that this writing will move many into action. Action that leads us to self awareness, self improvement, and helps us to realize that we have environmental responsibilities.

We are all a part of one. Whatever affects one has a corresponding effect on others. In nature the same is true. If we are responsible and respectful of our great mother she will pay us back tenfold. Isn't that a great return on our investment?

Recipes

"But the flesh with the life thereof which is the blood thereof, shall ye not eat." Genesis 9:4

The Quality Foods

This section contains fifty recipes that are great tasting and easy to prepare. The recipes are made with one-hundred percent all natural ingredients. No white flour, sugar, or animal products are used (except the vanilla cake in the dessert section contains eggs).

The great majority of the ingredients are fine for those who must be on special diets. People with diabetes, heart trouble, high blood pressure, and other health problems can enjoy the great majority of these recipes without health concerns. Even people on weight loss, weight gain or exercise (high carbohydrate) diets will find that these recipes will satisfy their requirements. However, we do ask you to carefully read the ingredients.

Cooking and preparing food can be very exciting, enriching and rewarding. It's important for all of us to eat balanced, quality meals. The recipes contained within would be a wonderful addition to your regular cooking regimen. And many can be prepared quickly.

Most of the recipes contained within were served at the Natural Oasis Vegetarian Restaurant in Philadelphia, Pennsylvania which I owned and operated. Many of the customers suggested that I have cooking classes to demonstrate how to prepare the food. The recipe section is the next best thing.

Feel free to try as many of the recipes as you desire. The directions are as clear and straight forward as possible. Not only are they delicious, but the nutrition standards are very high.

SALADS, RAW DISHES, AND VEGETABLE DISHES

CORN SALAD

2-3 ears corn, cut off the cob
¼ cup scallions, chopped
1 large stalk of celery, finely chopped
¼ cup tomato, finely chopped or
¼ cup red pepper
1 small carrot, finely grated
¼ cup broccoli, finely chopped (optional)
1 tsp. dried parsley
½ tsp. oregano
½ tsp. spike, vege-sal or herbamare
¼ cup eggless mayonnaise (or more to taste)

☞   Mix vegetables together. Add parsley, oregano, and spike (or other salt substitute) to vegetable mixture. Stir well. Add eggless mayonnaise. Blend well.

RED CABBAGE SALAD

1 small red cabbage, finely shredded
1 yellow onion, thinly sliced
1 cucumber, cut into thin strips
½ cup golden raisins (or regular raisins)
½ cup olive oil
¼ cup red wine vinegar
¼ cup finely chopped fresh dill
1 tablespoon lemon juice
1 tsp. sea salt
1 tsp. black pepper
1 green pepper cut into thin strips

☞   In large bowl, combine red cabbage, onion, cucumber, green peppers, and raisins. In small bowl, blend olive oil, vinegar, dill, lemon juice, salt, and pepper. Pour dressing over salad and toss well. Cover and refrigerate.

Time: Let stand about 2 hours to blend flavors.

COUNTRY COLESLAW

½ head red cabbage, shredded
½ head green cabbage, shredded
½ cup carrots, shredded
½ cup raisins
⅓ cup onion, finely chopped
1 tbsp. celery seeds

1 tsp. honey

2 tsp. lemon juice

½ cup eggless mayonnaise
¼ tsp. sea salt
dash of cayenne pepper

☞ Combine vegetables with raisins. Add spices and honey. Stir well. Add lemon juice and eggless mayonnaise. Blend well. Keep refrigerated until serving.

TOFU "EGGLESS" SALAD

1 lb. firm tofu
½ cup onions, finely chopped or
½ cup scallions, chopped
½ cup celery, finely chopped
1 green or red pepper, chopped
2 garlic cloves minced or 1 tsp. of garlic powder
1 small carrot, grated

¼ cup fresh parsley, chopped
1 ½ tsp. tumeric
1 tsp. Dr. Bronner's protein seasoning
1 tsp. tamari
1 ½ tsp. mustard
¼ cup eggless mayonnaise
1 tsp. nutritional yeast (optional)

☞ Mash tofu. Add vegetables and stir well. Add spices and mustard. Blend. Add tamari. Stir in eggless mayonnaise. Serve on bed of romaine lettuce, with a salad, or in pita bread.

MARINATED BEETS

5 small to medium-sized beets, scrubbed and sliced
1 small to medium-sized carrot (slivered)
1 small to medium-sized onion (sliced)
2 ½ tbsps. extra virgin olive oil
4 tbsps. freshly squeezed lemon juice
2 cloves garlic, minced
½ tsp. sea salt
3 tbsps. slivered scallions
Minced fresh parsley for garnish

☛   Mix vegetables together. Mix olive oil, lemon juice, garlic and sea salt until blended well. Pour olive oil mixture over vegetables and mix well. Let sit at least 6 hours at room temperature. Then serve. It is better to allow mixture to sit in refrigerator for 24 hours. Garnish with minced parsley before serving.

KUSH
(Very similar to Taboulli Salad)

1 cup cracked wheat (bulgur #1 or #2)
1 small carrot, finely grated
1 small onion, finely chopped or (1/4 cup scallions, finely chopped)
2 stalks celery, finely diced
½ green pepper, finely diced (optional)
2 cloves garlic, finely minced
2 tsp. sesame oil
1 tsp. tumeric or paprika
¼ cup fresh chopped parsley
2 tsp. tamari
1 tsp. sage
1 tsp. Dr. Bronner's protein seasoning
1 tsp. spike or vegesal
2 tsp. olive oil

☛   Place cracked wheat in medium-sized bowl. Add spices and stir well. Add ⅞ cup boiling water (use 1 cup boiling water if using bulgur #2). Cover and let sit for approximately 20-25 minutes or until grain is soft but chewy. Add tamari, vegetables and oil. Stir well. Chill in refrigerator until ready to serve.

TANGY TOFU DRESSING

2 square cakes of tofu (soft)
3 cloves garlic, diced
¼ cup oil
¼ cup tamari
¼ cup water
1 tbsp. parsley

2 tsp. thyme
1 ½ tsp. cayenne pepper
   (more or less depending on
   your taste)
juice of 1 lemon

☞   Slowly add all ingredients to blender. Blend until creamy smooth. Makes a very good salad dressing.

Variation: **You can add a few pieces of fresh spinach for color or a tomato for color and taste.**

GUACAMOLE D-LITE

2-3 medium avocados (make
   sure they are ripe)
1 ripe medium tomato
4 tbsp. minced onion
¾ tsp. garlic powder or 1
   clove garlic, minced

¾ tsp. sea salt or herbal seasoning
½ sp. chili powder
2 tbsp. fresh squeezed lemon
   juice (juice of ½ lemon)
½ tsp. tamari

☞   Cut avocados in half and scoop out inside and put seed aside. Mash the avocados. Peel and chop the tomato. Add tomato to mashed avocado mixture. Add the rest of the ingredients. Mix well. Replace seed in mixture if you do not plan to serve immediately. This will prevent mixture from turning brown. Refrigerate until ready to serve. Serve as dip with chips or in a sandwich.

DILLED GREEN BEANS

2 lbs green beans (or string beans)
Olive oil for sauteeing
1 tsp. dried dill

Vege-sal or other herbal seasoning to taste
Spring water

☞   Prepare green beans by breaking ends off and rinsing in cold water. Set aside. Place oil in pot over medium heat. Add string beans and stir continuously until beans are bright green. Add boiling water to cover. Simmer until tender. Add dill and vege-sal. Stir and serve.

SAUTEED CUCUMBERS

1 green onion (scallion) minced
3 tbsps. soy margarine

3 cucumbers, cut into ½ inch slices
Sea salt or vege-sal
Chopped dill

☞   Sauté the green onion in the margarine until limp. Add the sliced cucumbers and salt to taste. Cook on low heat, turning cucumbers frequently for 5 minutes, or until tender. Sprinkle with chopped dill and serve warm.

SAUTEED CABBAGE

1 medium head of cabbage, shredded	Oil
	Soy margarine
1 medium onion, diced	Vege-sal to taste
1 medium green pepper, sliced thin	Parsley, chopped
	1 clove garlic, minced
1 ½ tsp. turmeric	

☞   Add oil and soy margarine to pan. Then, add cabbage and other vegetables. Add turmeric, garlic, vege-sal and parsley. Stir frequently. Add a little water if veggies start to stick. Simmer on low until cabbage is tender and slightly crisp.

Variation: Also veggies can be sauteed with black mustard seeds.

SAVOY CABBAGE AND KALE

1 head savoy cabbage (can use green, red or Chinese cabbage)	Sesame seeds
	Tamari (optional)
	Soy margarine (optional)
1 bunch kale	1 clove garlic, diced

☞   Chop cabbage into bite-sized pieces. Chop kale. Steam cabbage and kale with garlic.* When vegetables are slightly tender, and bright green in color, turn off fire. Add sesame seeds. Serve with soy margarine and/or tamari.

*Kale and sesame seeds are both very good sources of calcium.

MACARONI SALAD

12 oz. box macaroni
  (Debole's macaroni works
  well)
½ cup carrots, shredded
⅓ cup bell pepper, chopped
½ cup celery, chopped
1 clove garlic, minced
1 tsp. sea salt
2 tsp. vege-sal (or to taste)

2 tsp. dried parsley
A dash of cayenne pepper
1 cup soy mayonnaise
1 cup firm tofu, cubed
3 tbsps. relish
1 tomato, diced (optional)
a cup scallions sliced (or
  chopped onions)

☛   Cook macaroni according to directions. Allow to cool. Mix all ingredients well. Keep refrigerated until serving time.

CARROT TUNA

2 tsp. carrot juice
Carrot pulp (leftover from
  freshly juiced carrot juice)
¼ cup onions (or 2 scallions
  diced in small pieces)
1 stalk celery, diced in small
  pieces
Eggless mayonnaise to taste

¼ tsp. spike, herbamare, or
  other herbal seasoning
¼ tsp. lemon juice
1 tbsp. tamari
1 tsp. dill
1 tsp. parsley
Sea salt (optional)
Relish (optional)

☛   Juice carrots and remove pulp from juicer. (Use good juicer to insure pulp will be dry), clean pulp (remove particles that are large or discolored). Fluff pulp with your fingers to make it flaky. Add vegetables. Add spike or other herbal seasoning, lemon juice, tamari, dill, parsley, sea salt (optional), and carrot juice. Blend well. Add eggless mayonnaise and blend well. Serve on bed of Romaine or in Pita bread.

SOUPS

CREAM OF BROCCOLI SOUP

1 Bunch broccoli
¼ cup arrowroot flour
½ tsp. garlic powder
1 tsp. onion powder

1 tbsp. vegetable powder
16 oz. soy milk
½ cup soy margarine
⅓ cup water

☞   Chop broccoli and cook in water. Then pour ½ of cooked broccoli and remainder of cooking water into the blender. Blend until broccoli is creamed. In a heavy saucepan, melt ¼ cup soy margarine and remainder of ingredients. Cook slowly, add more milk until soup is a creamy consistency. Add remainder of soy margarine last.

SPLIT PEA SOUP

1 ½ cups green split peas, rinsed and sorted
6 cups cold water
1 medium-sized onion, chopped
2 carrots, chopped
2 ribs celery, chopped
1 tsp. salt

1 tsp. Dr. Bronner's protein seasoning
1 tsp. garlic powder
½ tsp. thyme
Pinch of cayenne
2 tsps. parsley
2 tbsps. nutritional yeast
1 tbsp. tamari

☞   In large soup pot, add peas and *cold* water. Simmer until peas are soft but not mushy. Add vegetables. Simmer until vegetables are soft and soup is creamy. Add seasonings and tamari. Simmer another 10 minutes.

NAVY BEAN SOUP

1 lb. navy beans, rinsed and
   sorted
8 cups water
1 large onion, chopped
4 stalks celery, chopped
celery leaves, chopped
2 cups tomatoes chopped

½ tsp. sea salt, vege-sal or
   other herbal seasoning
2 tbsp. olive oil
1 tsp. parsley
2 tsp. tamari
¼ tsp. cayenne pepper

☛   Start beans to cook in cold water under low heat. Once beans are tender add vegetables. Simmer until vegetables are soft. Make sure beans are still firm but tender. Add tamari. Add oil, celery leaves, parsley, and sea salt. Simmer for approx. 10 minutes more or until flavors blend. Add tomatoes. Simmer for another 5 minutes. Serve warm and enjoy.

VEGETABLE BARLEY SOUP

¾ cup yellow squash, diced
1 tsp. safflower oil
1 cup chopped onion
1 cup carrot, sliced thinly
1 cup celery sliced
1 tbsp. minced garlic
2 cups tomatoes, chopped
1 cup barley

1 tsp. parsley
1 tsp. thyme
1 tsp. oregano
6 cups soup stock or water
1 tsp. vege-sal or other herbal
   seasoning
1 ½ tsp. tamari

☛   In large soup pot, heat oil and sauté onion until soft but not brown. To keep onion from sticking, add water as needed. Add remaining vegetables, herbs, tamari, and barley. Sauté for approx. 8-10 minutes. Add stock or water and bring to a boil. Lower heat, cover, and simmer soup (until barley is tender), approximately 45 minutes. Taste, and adjust seasoning and serve warm.

MINESTRONE SOUP

2 cups cooked kidney beans
2 onions, chopped
4 stalks of celery, chopped
4 carrots, sliced
1 small cabbage shredded
1-2 medium red (new)
    potatoes, chopped
Safflower oil
4 cups tomatoes chopped
2 tsp. garlic powder
2 tsp. oregano

4 tsp. basil
2 tsp. sea salt
½ tsp. pepper or herbal
    seasoning
1 tbsp. dried parsley
8 cups water
1 cup cooked macaroni noo-
    dles (Debole's works well).
2 tbsp. tamari

☞   Sauté onions, celery, carrots, cabbage, and potatoes in oil until tender. Next add remaining ingredients except for tomatoes, noodles and beans. Allow this to come to a boil. Boil for 15 minutes, stirring occasionally to keep from sticking. Add the beans, 1 cup noodles, and tomatoes and simmer for a few minutes before serving.

LENTIL SOUP

2 cups lentils
6 cups cold water or cold
    soup stock
1 large onion, chopped
2 carrots, diced
½ cup celery diced

1 clove garlic, minced
2 tsps. dried parsley
2 tbsps. tamari
2 tsps. vege-sal or herbal
    seasoning
2 tsps. olive oil

☞   In large pot, simmer lentils in cold water until almost done (soft but not mushy). Add vegetables. Simmer until vegetables are soft. Add parsley, oil, tamari, and herbal seasonings. Simmer approximately another 5-10 minutes until flavors are blended well.

ENTREES AND SANDWICHES

RATATOUILLE
(Eggplant Casserole)

1 eggplant, cubed (peeling
  the skin is optional)
1 onion, chopped
2 green peppers, chopped
4 zucchini, cubed
5 tomatoes, chopped
2 tbsps. olive oil

2 cloves garlic, chopped
2 tbsps. fresh parsley
1 tsp. oregano
Soy margarine for sauteeing
Optional: ½ cup Soy
  Parmesan Cheese, grated

☛   In large skillet, sauté eggplant in oil and margarine until tender. Add onions, peppers, and zucchini. Stir until vegetables are tender. Add tomatoes and seasonings. Place mixture in an oiled baking dish. Sprinkle with grated soy cheese (optional).

Time: Bake at 325º for 15 minutes. Serve over brown rice or millet.

SUCCOTASH

5 ears yellow corn
½ pound okra
3 medium tomatoes chopped
½ cup safflower oil

2 medium onions
½ tsp. salt
⅛ tsp. black pepper

☛   Into large bowl, cut corn from cob. Cut twice, scraping cob with knife to get "milk". Trim ends from okra and cut into 1 inch thick slices. In large skillet, heat oil, add okra and onions. Cook on medium heat stirring occasionally, until onion is transparent. Stir in corn, season with salt and pepper. Cook on medium-high heat, stirring occasionally about 20 minutes. Lower heat. Add tomatoes, cover and cook for another 5 minutes.

BROWN RICE AND VEGETABLES

1 cup brown rice	1 cup of chopped broccoli
2 tbsp. of sesame oil	1 medium onion, sliced thinly
2 tbsp. of tamari	1 cup of mushrooms (sliced)
2 cups of water	1 medium zucchini or yellow
1 tablespoon of vegetable	squash, slice diagonally
powder	2 tsp. oil to add to rice
1 carrot, sliced thinly	

☞   Wash rice and put it in a small saucepan. Add 2 tsp. oil, tamari, and vegetable powder. Mix well and add 2 cups water. Cook on medium fire for 45 minutes. Place 2 tablespoons of sesame oil in wok. Add all vegetables to wok and stir fry until tender. Then add vegetable mixture to cooked rice.

SCRAMBLED TOFU

1 medium onion, finely	1 tbsp. tamari
chopped	½ tsp. tumeric
1 lb. firm tofu (crumbled)	2 tbsp. safflower oil or
½ tsp. spike	1 tbsp. soy margarine
1 tsp. nutritional yeast flakes	

☞   Sauté onions in oil for 5-10 minutes. Add crumbled tofu and stir well.* Add yeast flakes, spike, tamari, and turmeric. Simmer for another 10-15 minutes. This dish resembles scrambled eggs and is a delicious breakfast food.

*Optional - Add 1 medium green pepper, chopped.

BAKED BEANS

1 lb. dried navy beans, rinsed and sorted
1 - 6 oz. can tomato paste or tomato sauce
1 tbsp. tamari sauce
¼ tsp. dry mustard

½ tsp. garlic powder
½ cup chopped onion
½ cup chopped green pepper
¼ cup raw honey
2 tbsp. pure molasses
¼ cup margarine

☛   Wash beans. Place beans in cold water and bring to a boil. Allow to simmer until tender, approximately 1-½ hours. Add remaining ingredients. Pour beans and ingredients in a large baking dish. Bake for 2 hrs. at 300°. Serves four.

TOFU RICE CROQUETTES

1 medium onion, finely diced
1 cup celery or green pepper, finely diced
1 small carrot, finely grated
½ cup sunflower seeds (or almonds, walnuts, or pumpkin seeds)
¾ cup cooked brown rice
⅓ cup rolled oats
1 ½ cup whole wheat bread crumbs
1 ½ pound mashed tofu (use firm tofu)

¼ cup chopped fresh parsley (2 tbsps. if dried)
2 tbsps. ketchup
1 ½ tsp. thyme
1 tsp. vege-sal or spike
1 tbsp. tamari sauce
1 tsp. garlic powder (or 2 cloves fresh garlic)
2 tsp. nutritional yeast
1 tsp Dr. Bronner's protein seasoning

☛   Grind seeds or nuts. Mix all ingredients in a large bowl. Let sit about ½ hour. Shape into croquettes. Bake in oiled pan. Bake until golden brown. This mixture can also be baked in a loaf pan.

SUMMER SQUASH MEDLEY

3 medium-sized summer squash, sliced or cut into chunks	1 tsp. tamari
	1 clove garlic (minced)
	2 tsp. parsley
1 onion thinly sliced	oil for sauteeing
1 medium tomato chopped	Add vegesal to taste

☞　　Sauté onion and squash in oil. Add a small amount of water to allow vegetables to steam. Cover and cook until tender. Add vegesal, tamari, garlic, tomatoes and parsley. Simmer for another 5 minutes. Serve warm. Can also be used with green zucchini.

SLOPPY JOES

1 cup dry T.V.P.	½ tsp. basil
1 tbsp. vegetable oil	½ tsp. parsley
½ large onion, chopped	1 cup tomato sauce
½ green pepper, chopped	1 tbsp. chili powder
2 cloves garlic, diced	½ tsp. oregano
¼ tsp. sea salt	

☞　　Hydrate T.V.P. by adding ⅞ cup boiling water to 1 cup dry T.V.P. Sauté onion, green pepper and garlic in oil for approximately 3-4 minutes. Add hydrated T.V.P., sea salt, chili powder and herbs. Stir and blend well. Add tomato sauce. Simmer on medium low heat for approximately 10 minutes until vegetables are tender. Serve on whole wheat buns or toasted English muffins.

Variation:　　½ lb. firm tofu can be substituted for T.V.P. Mash tofu to crumbly consistency.

SPICY CARROTS

1 lb. bag fresh carrots, cut
   into 1" chunks
1 ½ tsp. cinnamon
1 ½ tsp. allspice seasoning

1 tsp. curry powder
¼ cup water
½ stick soy margarine

☛   Bring water to boil in a medium-sized pot. Add carrots. Mix spices and add to pot. Cook at medium high temperature for 5 minutes. Add soy margarine. Cook at medium temperature for another 5 minutes.

VEGETARIAN CHOW MEIN

4 tbsps. safflower oil
3 cups firm tofu, cut into
   cubes
1 medium onion, sliced
2 large bell peppers, cut into
   strips
6 stalks celery, sliced
   diagonally

½ cup water
⅓ cup tamari
½ tsp. garlic powder (or 1
   clove of garlic minced)
2 cups mung bean sprouts
½ lb. fresh mushrooms, sliced

☛   Heat oil in skillet. Add tofu and cook over medium low heat until the cubes are browned. Stir occasionally to brown all sides of the cubes. Add vegetables except mushrooms and sprouts. Cover and simmer for 5 minutes. Stir several times. Combine water, tamari, and garlic. Mix well and pour over tofu and vegetables. Continue cooking at low heat for another 10-15 minutes. During the last 5 minutes, add sprouts and mushrooms. Serve over brown rice.

STUFFED PEPPERS

Medium bell peppers (2
   per person)
1 small onion, chopped
3 stalks celery, chopped
10 mushrooms, sliced
2 cups cooked rice tomato
   sauce or spaghetti sauce
(to desired consistency)

2 tbsps. vegetable oil
1 ½ cups cooked beans
   (pintos, red, lentil, or black)
1 cup soy cheese, grated
vege-sal, spike, or herbamare
   to taste
parsley

☛   Wash peppers. Remove stem and seeds. In large pot, boil peppers. Remove from pot and allow peppers to cool. In large skillet, sauté onion, celery, and mushrooms in oil. Add rice, tomato sauce, beans, parsley, and seasoning. Simmer a few minutes. Fill peppers with rice mixture and place them on cookie sheet. Sprinkle with soy cheese.

Time: Bake at 350º for approximately 20 minutes or until cheese melts.

PITA PIZZA

Pita Bread
Spaghetti or Pizza Sauce
Grated tofu mozzarella
   cheese
Fresh vegetables such as:

Sliced mushrooms
Grated carrots
Chopped onions
Chopped green pepper, etc.
Oregano (optional)

☛   Spread sauce on pita bread. Add grated cheese. Arrange vegetables on pita in a decorative manner. Sprinkle on oregano.

Time: Bake in oven at 350º for about 15 minutes or until cheese melts.

VEGGIES-N-PITA

Lettuce
Spinach
1 stalk celery
½ small cucumber
1 small carrot
2 cups alfalfa sprouts

½ avocado
1-2 tbsps. eggless mayonnaise
*½ tsp. mustard
fresh lemon juice
sea salt
2 whole wheat pitas

☛   Finely chop lettuce, spinach, celery, and cucumber. Combine in a small bowl. Grate carrot and dice avocado. Mix vegetables and sprouts. Next, add mayonnaise and mustard with a squeeze of lemon juice and sea salt to taste. Mix well. Stuff salad mixture into pita pockets.

*Tamari can be substituted for mustard. Also chopped tomato can be added if you plan to eat it immediately.

SEITAN PEPPER STEAK

16 oz. seitan (wheat gluten)
½ cup green pepper, sliced
   in strips
½ cup onions, sliced thin
½ tsp. basil
½ tsp. parsley

¼ tsp. spike
2 tbsps. safflower oil
½ cup water
½ tsp. honey
1 tsp. arrowroot flour
2 tbsps. tamari

☛   Slice seitan into narrow strips. Sprinkle with spike and set aside. Prepare vegetables. Add oil, basil, parsley, and seitan, and vegetables in a wok. Allow vegetables to steam until tender. Then mix honey, tamari, arrowroot flour, and water together. Pour over vegetables and seitan. Let it simmer 5 minutes. Serve over brown rice.

VEGETABLE STEW WITH SEITAN

1 container of seitan, chopped (approx. 14-16 oz)
3 medium sized carrots, sliced
1 large onion chopped
2 stalks celery, sliced
2 ears of corn, (removed from the cob)
4 potatoes cubed (with skin)
2 large bell peppers, chopped
1 cup broccoli flowerettes

1 yellow squash, sliced or chopped
1 clove of garlic, minced
2 vegetable bouillon cubes
3 tomatoes, chopped
1 ½ tbsp tamari
½ tsp. sea salt or herbal seasoning
2 tsp. basil
2 tsp. parsley
2 tsp. vegetable oil

☛ Scrub potatoes and boil until tender but not too soft. Set potatoes aside. Fry seitan in vegetable oil and set aside. Add all of the remaining ingredients (except broccoli and tomatoes) to a large pot with about 10 cups of water. Cook under a medium flame. When everything has cooked for approximately 20 minutes, add seitan, broccoli, and potatoes and cook for another 5-10 minutes so mixture can blend. Add tomatoes after stew is finished cooking.

BLUEBERRY YAMS

5 large sweet potatoes, sliced
¾ cup raisins
1 ½ cup blueberries
1 tsp. allspice seasoning

1 tbsp. cinnamon
1 stick of Soy margarine
¼ cup of honey

☛ Cover the bottom of casserole dish with 2 layers of sweet potatoes. Add layer of blueberries and raisins proportionally. Repeat, starting with one layer of sweet potatoes. Mix allspice and cinnamon and drizzle on top. Top with soy margarine and a thin glaze of honey. Cook until potatoes are soft.

VEGETARIAN LASAGNA

Spaghetti sauce with T.V.P
  (textured vegetable
  protein)
1 box lasagna
¾ lb. tofu

⅓ lbs. thinly sliced tofu mozzarella cheese
½ lbs. soy cheese, grated

☛   Prepare lasagna, and set aside. Pre-heat oven to 350°. Spread a thin layer of sauce in a baking dish. Add a layer of lasagna noodles. Cover with a sprinkle of the cheese and tofu. Cover with another layer of sauce. Then another layer of pasta and a layer of tofu and cheeses. Continue to build layers reserving enough sauce to cover final layer of pasta. Cover final layer of pasta with tofu mozzarella cheese.

Time: Bake 30-40 minutes. Let stand briefly before cutting and serving.

SPICY PINTO BEAN STEW

1 lb. pinto beans
1 large onion, chopped
1 green bell pepper, chopped
2 tsp. black pepper
8 oz. tomato paste
2 cloves garlic, diced

¼ cup vegetable oil
2 tsp. vege-sal
2 tsp. hot sauce
¾ cup Dr. Bronner's
  Balanced Mineral Bouillon
6 cups cold water

☛   Cook beans in cold water until halfway done. Should be approximately 40-60 minutes. Then add onion, green pepper, garlic, vegetable oil. Add rest of ingredients (except Dr. Bronner's). Resume cooking for another 40 minutes or until beans are tender at medium temperature. When beans are done, add Dr. Bronner's and more water if needed for stew-like consistency. Stir for 1 minute, serve warm with hot corn bread muffins.

SEITAN "STEAKWICH" WITH CHEESE

1 container (approx. 14-16   2 tsp. Tamari
  oz) Seitan, sliced   1 tsp. Nutritional yeast flakes
1 medium onion, sliced   Oil
1 medium green bell pepper,   Grated soy cheese (optional)
  in strips

☛   Sauté seitan with onions in oil. Add strips of green pepper. Add tamari and nutritional yeast flakes. When seitan is done. Add grated soy cheese. Cover and simmer until cheese is melted. Serve on a whole wheat bun with the "works".

SPAGHETTI SAUCE WITH T.V.P.

½ cup celery, chopped   ½ tsp. basil
1 cup onion, chopped   1/4 tsp. thyme
½ cup green pepper,   ½ tsp. oregano
  chopped   ½ tsp. chives
1 garlic clove, minced   1 tsp. parsley
1 cup mushrooms, sliced   1 cup textured vegetable
2 tbsps. olive oil   protein (T.V.P)
1 small jar spaghetti sauce   ⅞ cup water (boiled)
1-6 oz. can tomato paste   1 lb. spaghetti (either whole
6 oz. water   wheat or other type)
1 tbsp. tamari sauce

☛   Pour olive oil in a large iron skillet. Sauté garlic first, then add onion, green pepper, celery, and mushrooms. Next, add the basil, thyme, oregano, chives, and parsley. Let it simmer. Meanwhile, put the T.V.P in a bowl with the boiling water. Let it set for about 15 minutes. Next, add the tomato paste slowly into the vegetable mixture with 6 oz. of water. Stir in spaghetti sauce. Add tamari last. Allow to simmer on low heat. Prepare spaghetti as package indicates. Drain well. Add the T.V.P to the spaghetti sauce and mix well. Pour over spaghetti as you desire.

DESSERTS, BREADS, AND BEVERAGES

APPLE CRISP

1 ⅓ cup rolled oats
⅔ cup whole wheat pastry
    flour
1 pinch sea salt and 1/8 tsp.
    sea salt
⅓ cup soy margarine,
    melted
⅓ cup honey or blueberry
    syrup

⅔ cup chopped walnuts (or
    any nuts)
¼ cup apple juice
½ tbsp. lemon juice
2 tsps. vanilla
1 tsp. cinnamon
5 cups chopped apples
¾ cup raisins or blueberries
¼ tsp. nutmeg

☞   Preheat oven to 350⁰. Mix flour, oats, and ⅛ tsp. salt. Then drizzle in margarine and mix well. Add ⅓ cup honey and mix well. Then mix in nuts. Dissolve a pinch of salt in ¼ cup apple juice. Add vanilla, lemon juice and spices. Mix well, then toss with apples and raisins. Next place apple mixture in a buttered 8"x8" baking pan. Lightly spoon topping over apple mixture.

Time: Bake 45 minutes until topping is golden brown and crispy.

CORN BREAD MUFFINS

1 cup whole wheat flour (or
    soy flour)
1 cup cornmeal
¼ cup honey
2 tsp. baking powder

1 cup soy milk
⅓ cup melted soy margarine
    or oil
¼ cup water

☞   Combine flour, cornmeal, and baking powder in a medium-size bowl. Combine soy margarine and honey in a separate bowl. Then, add to flour mixture and blend well. Add soy milk, water, and blend well.

Time: Bake in oiled muffin pans at 350⁰ for approximately 20-25 minutes.

APPLESAUCE CAKE

½ cup chopped apples
½ cup raisins
1 cup honey
½ cup oil
1 ½ cups unsweetened
    applesauce

2 cups whole wheat flour
½ tsp. salt
1 ½ tsp. baking powder
1 tsp. cinnamon
½ tsp. nutmeg

☞   In large bowl, beat honey and oil until smooth. Add apple-sauce and mix in the dry ingredients. Blend well until smooth. Pour batter into oiled 8" cake pan or loaf pan. Bake in preheated oven (350º) for 45-50 minutes. This cake is even better the next day.

OATMEAL RAISIN COOKIES

½ cup raisins
3 cups rolled oats
1 tsp. salt (sea salt)
2 tsp. baking powder
2 ½ cups whole wheat pastry
    flour

2 tsp. vanilla
⅓ cup soy milk
1 cup honey
⅓ cup oil
½ cup margarine

Cream margarine, oil, and honey together. Add soy milk and vanilla. Beat until smooth. Beat in flour, salt, and baking powder. Mix, add oats and raisins, and blend well. Bake at 350º for about 15 minutes.

FRUIT NUT BALLS

1 cup dates (pitted)
1 cup ground Brazil nuts
½ cup ground almonds
½ cup dried pineapple,
  chopped
½ cup dried papaya,
  chopped

½ tsp. cinnamon
½ tsp. nutmeg
Dried coconut
½ cup raisins (soft)

☛   Add nuts to food processor. Add fruit and spices. Blend well. Roll mixture in coconut and form into balls. Allow to set in refrigerator to harden. Wrap in wax paper to store.

VANILLA CAKE WITH CREAMY CAROB ICING

¾ cup soy margarine
1 ¼ cup honey
2 eggs
1 ½ tsp. vanilla
3 cups sifted whole wheat
  flour

1 ½ tsp. baking powder
1 tsp. salt (sea salt)
¾ cup soy milk

☛   Preheat oven to 350⁰. Cream margarine and honey. Add eggs and vanilla and beat until fluffy. Sift dry ingredients together. Add creamed mixture alternately with milk, beating after each addition. Beat 1 minute. Bake in 2 greased and lightly floured round cake pans. Bake at 350⁰ for 30-35 minutes. Cool for 10 minutes before removing from the pans. Finish cooling before icing with the creamy carob icing. (Creamy Carob Icing on next page.)

CREAMY CAROB ICING

4 tsp. honey   **Soy milk (Edensoy)**
4 tbsp. carob powder   **1 tsp. vanilla**

☛   Mix carob powder with honey and vanilla. Blend well. Add enough soy milk to thin out frosting until desired consistency. (Can be used on any kind of cakes.)

PINA COLADA SMOOTHIE

1 ½ cup coconut milk   **1 banana (frozen or fresh)**
1 cup pineapple juice   **Honey or maple syrup to taste**
½ cup strawberries (frozen
**   or fresh)**

☛   Blend until mixed well. If frozen fruit is used, you may be able to eliminate or decrease the amount of honey or maple syrup used.

LOCAL NUTRI SMOOTHIE

1 pint of natural apple juice
1 banana
5 small strawberries

1 scoop of C.C.I.'s Bahamian Diet, Spiru-Tein or other nutrition supplement Connection or Stay Fit.

☞   Put in blender and blend for about 1 minute. Serve cold. If the fruit is frozen the smoothie will taste sweeter. Otherwise add honey to taste.

POWER PUNCH SMOOTHIE

2 cups apple juice
1 frozen medium size banana
Handful of berries (strawberries or blueberries) can be fresh or frozen.

1 tsp. wheat germ (high in Vitamin E)
1 tsp. grounded sesame seeds (high in calcium and protein)
Honey or maple syrup to taste

☞   Blend all ingredients until mixture is mixed well. Optional, any of the following can be added to make this a very nutritious and powerful drink. Can add fresh bee pollen (½ tsp.), lecithin granules (1 tsp.), foods formula of the CCI's supplements or Nu-Plus whole food concentrate.

CAROB PUDDING

½ cup raisins
2 pitted dates
⅓ cup raw almonds
5 tablespoons unsweetened
  carob powder

1 ¼ cup carob (or vanilla)
  soymilk
2 or 3 ripe bananas (frozen
  will be sweeter)

☛   Put ingredients into blender and blend for 2 minutes. Serve at room temperature or refrigerate for 1 hour if desired. If you desire a thicker consistency, add more almonds or raisins as desired. If you desire a thinner consistency, add more soymilk as desired. (Makes 3 to 5 servings)

HELPFUL HINTS

1. *Nutritional yeast* adds a cheesy taste to vegetarian dishes. It also is a good source of B vitamins.

2. *Brags liquid aminos* is a substitute for tamari for those on salt-restricted diets. It is also a good source of protein.

3. *Soybeans* are used to make many products that are meatless and good sources of protein. Tofu, tempeh, textured vegetable protein (T.V.P), nuts, margarine, milk, flour, oil, soy sauce, and miso are just a few of the products made from soybeans.

4. *Tofu* is a complete source of protein. It has a bland taste and will mix well with any food. It should also have a bland, non-offensive smell when you are purchasing it. Try to buy it fresh from a bulk supply rather than packaged. It will usually have a fresher taste. Tofu should also be kept in water and stored in a covered container. The water should be changed daily in order to maintain freshness.

5. When using T.V.P (textured vegetable protein), add 7/8 cup boiling water to 1 cup of dry T.V.P to yield 2 cups of hydrated T.V.P. T.V.P has the shape and texture of hamburger and can be used as a substitute for hamburger in recipes.

6. *Homemade bread crumbs* can be made by toasting whole wheat bread and dicing it into bite-size pieces. Allow the bread crumbs to sit out overnight.

7. *Brown rice* is more nutritious than white rice. In the process of making white rice, the brown outer covering is removed and the white inner grain is polished. This process cuts the fiber content by 2/3 and removes a large portion of the vitamins and minerals.

8. *Perfect brown rice* is made by rinsing first in cold water and cooking it in cold water. Add seasonings first, add 1 tsp. oil and 2 cups of cold water for each cup of rice. Bake at 350° until the water is absorbed.

9. *Cayenne pepper* is good to add to foods. It helps to stimulate the digestive process. Also garlic and ginger are good to use.

10. When cooking legumes, you do not need to soak peas and lentils. Also most other beans (except soy beans and chickpeas) do not need to be soaked if you start them to cook in cold water. You may soak the beans overnight but most times it is

not necessary. Also, cooking beans in a slow cooker (or crock pot) will yield very tender beans and will also decrease preparation time.

11. Cooking in cast iron pots and pans will increase the iron content of foods.

12. *Carob* can be used instead of chocolate. Carob is an excellent source of calcium. It is also called St. John's Bread. It contains no chocolate, caffeine, or cocoa.

13. When a recipe calls for honey, add oil to the measuring cup first. The honey will pour our easily.

14. To obtain a non-stick coating on a baking pan, use 2 parts lecithin to 1 part oil.

15. Sea kelp and dulse, 2 types of seaweeds, are very nice sources of necessary minerals and they are highly alkaline. They can be used as a salt substitute and added to salads, soups, stews, rice, or steamed veggies.

16. *Arrowroot flour* can be used in place of cornstarch to thicken fruits, soups, and gravy. Add 1 cup water to 1 ½ tbsp. arrowroot. Bring to a boil to thicken.

17. Mix nuts and raisins with dry ingredients to keep from sinking to bottom of bowl.

18. Leftover foods are best stored in glass jars to prevent them from picking up or giving off odors.

19. Millet is an alkaline grain. To cook, add 2 cups water to 1 cup millet and 1 vegetable bouillon cube or tamari to taste. Cook until water is absorbed over medium heat. Watch carefully because millet cooks fast.

20. Good oils to use are safflower, sunflower, corn, olive, soy, sesame, or canola oils. Avoid palm oils, palm kernel oils and coconut oils for they are high in unsaturated fats.

21. Wheat germ is high in protein, B vitamins, vitamin E, potassium, and zinc.

22. Add 1 tbsp. of oil to pasta while it is cooking to prevent it from boiling over or sticking together.

23. There are commercial products such as Ener-G Egg Replacer which can be used in place of eggs in recipes. Other substitutes are:

a) ½ tsp. each arrowroot and soy flour mixed in 2 cups warm water.

b) ½ tsp. lecithin per lb. of batter.

c) ⅛ banana mashed

d) ⅛ tofu blended with liquid

Also sometimes you don't need to use the substitute because the egg can be eliminated from the recipe.

24. Remember to collect any recipes that you may like, even if they have to be adapted.

25. Rich sources of calcium are leafy green vegetables (especially turnip, collard, and mustard greens, kale, and broccoli); legumes (black-eyed peas, kidney beans, black beans, pinto beans, and soy beans); seeds (sesame seeds, sunflower seeds); dried fruit (dates, figs); and nut (almonds); molasses, and carob powder.

26. Debole's substitute pasta products are very good to use, especially if you want your recipe to resemble the "real" thing. These pasta products are made from semolina flour and American (Jerusalem) artichoke flour.

27. When a recipe calls for sugar: Replace 1 cup of sugar with ¾ cup of honey. Reduce liquid in recipe by ¼

28. DO NOT use aluminum cooking ware since aluminum can be absorbed into the body and can be a factor in causing alzheimer's disease.

29. Agar-Agar can be used as a jelling agent in place of animal gelatin. It jells readily at room temperature.

30. Try to prepare food with three goals in mind, namely, adequate nutritional value, an appetizing appearance, and a satisfying taste. Remember the first goal should be the most important.

SUGGESTED NATURAL FOODS

Fruits:

Apples	Apricots
Avocados	Bananas
Blackberries	Blueberries
Cantaloupe	Cherries
Cranberries	Currants
Figs (fresh)	Dates
Grapes	Grapefruits
Honeydew Melon	Guavas
Limes	Lemons
Nectarines	Mangoes
Papayas	Oranges
Pears	Peaches
Pineapples	Persimmons
Pomegranates	Plums
Raisins	Prunes
Strawberries	Raspberries
Watermelon	Tangerines

Vegetables:

AlfalfaSprouts	Artichokes (Jerusalem)
Asparagus	Bean Sprouts (all types)
Broccoli	Bok Choy
Beets	Cabbage (green or red)
Brussel Sprouts	Carrots
Cauliflower	Celery
Chinese Cabbage	Chives
Collards	Corn
Cucumbers	Dandelion Greens
Dill	Endive
Garlic	Green Beans
Green Peas	Green Peppers
Kale	Leeks
Lettuce (all types)	Mung Bean Sprouts
Mushrooms	Mustard Greens
Okra	Onions
Parsley	Parsnips

Potatoes

Red Peppers

Spinach

Swiss Chard

Tomatoes

Watercress

Radishes

Scallions

Squash-soft summer
 varieties

Turnip (green or tops)

Yams

Grains:

Whole Wheat

Cracked Wheat

Rye

Barley

Buckwheat

Kasha

Millet

Oats

Rice

Corn Flour

Soy Flour

Amaranth

Legumes:

Soybeans

Garbanzos (chick peas)

Split Peas

Lentils

Lima Beans

Navy Beans

Peas

Dried Beans

Mung Beans

Blackeyed Peas

Nuts and Seeds:

Almonds

Pumpkin Seeds

Cashews

Sunflower Seeds

Brazil Nuts

Sesame Seeds

Coconuts

Hazel Nuts (fiberts)

Walnuts

Dried fruits should be unsulfured. Watch food combinations:
Do not combine Fruits with vegetables, grains or legumes.

Wholistic Reflections

"Physicians Heal Thyselves"

Reviews

One of the purposes of this writing is to open our minds to new ideas with respect to diet and lifestyle. We wanted to properly explain the wholistic and vegetarian lifestyle to those who are just beginning to change their diet. We wanted to broaden the perspective and increase the knowledge of those who have already been on the road for a while. We all want positiveness, health, and tranquillity while living. This lifestyle is the most logical and viable means to achieving it.

Vegetarianism is a continuum in the knowledge of how to eat (and live). There are various degrees or levels of attainment. The first level of the transition is a lacto-ovo vegetarian (consumes dairy products, some white flour products but no red meat or any other animal flesh). The strict vegetarian who eats no animal products, no dairy, sugar, or flesh of any kind and practices good common sense eating habits. The next level is a raw food vegetarian who consumes no cooked food but mostly fruits, nuts, grains, vegetables, and legumes. The next level is a fruitatarian, who consumes only fruit. The final stage is a breathatarian, who consumes no food or juice. The breathatarian lives on fresh air, sunshine and a little water.

It may seem impractical but yes there are a few people in the world who don't eat for years and are strong, mentally sharp and in excellent health. Breathatarianism is not a realistic goal for most of us, but the higher that we elevate ourselves the more benefits we can attain.

There are people in India, China, and right here in America who are breathatarians. But they can only live in the rural areas and in the mountain areas where the air is pure and there is no man-made confusion. Some of the benefits of this lifestyle are clear thought, great discipline, self-control, and a tremendous potential for high spiritual understanding. We all need these benefits so let's help each other to get as much as we can (and more). Then we can be assured of our optimum state of well being.

The other main objectives of this writing were to substantiate that the body is not difficult to understand, that there are a variety of choices in producing wellness, and that you must play a part in staying healthy.

A physician or other health professional should almost be able to assure you of wellness if you follow the advice that they give. No health professional can absolutely guarantee wellness. But they should operate under ethical standards of sincerity and honesty when treating illness and/or promoting wellness. Additionally, they should have a good understanding of what it takes to be well physically, mentally, and spiritually. In other words, they should treat the whole person, not just a symptom of a problem.

I know many health professionals who do this, including several physicians. One doctor I know told me he doesn't need malpractice insurance because of the type of relationship that he has with his patients. He also doesn't prescribe drugs. He uses herbs, vitamins, and homeopathic medicines.

Herbs are nature's medicine for the great majority of people who have used them. Herbs have proven to be effective. That goes without saying when you consider that herbs have been used for medicinal purposes and health enhancement since the beginning of time. We just need to get back in touch with ourselves and the earth to experience the fullness and the abundance of life and all that it offers. No one said it is easy to do this but it's not that difficult. Besides our backs are against the wall and our great mother's karmic retribution is looking us right in the face. The opportunity to improve is in our hands.

We are created in the image and likeness of Almighty God. Within all of us is that great essence just waiting to be developed. Our desire should include its development.

We should be convinced that within each of us are the seeds of perfection. It is our right to grow and get some of that perfection. Maybe we can't get all of it, but we are entitled to all that we desire.

The wise and righteous mentalities of the past (Moses, Abraham, Solomon, Noah, Lot, and others) lived to be 150 to 950 years old. They ate very wholesomely and wisely. They didn't drink, smoke, or operate under negative emotions (e.g. frustration) for long periods of time.

It would be very difficult for us to live for hundreds of years. We have ill-treated ourselves and our environment excessively. We are under too much stress and are surrounded by negativity.

We are created perfect physically. Our challenge is to duplicate that perfection on a higher, spiritual plane. But we can't grow to that plane while we are eating wrong foods, taking drugs, cursing, etc. We can't grow if we are full of jealousy, hatred, and resentment. In other words, heaven and hell is a state of being that begins with our deeds, thoughts, and aspirations. So why don't we choose the best? Our great mother will nourish us and cherish us if we do.

It says in scripture that if you take the first steps toward improvement, the Creative Force will help and assist you. We must move on, evolve, grow and be like a tree. A tree grows and gets nourishment from the ground (earth) and from the sunlight (heaven) through the branches and leaves. We must eat wholesome nutritious foods to satisfy the lower self (earth). Our minds must be molded to receive the higher life from the heavenly sunshine of the presence of Almighty God.

Our Great Father (Almighty God) and our Great Mother (His Earthly Manifestation) do make us a promise. They promise us that if we adhere to the proper laws and rules for living on earth and use that guidance as a basis for developing our higher selves, we will have abundance, success, peace, and wellness. And that's a guarantee with everlasting implications.

Good fortune and many successes.

Selected Bibliography

KLOSS, JETHRO; *Back to Eden,* Back to Eden Books, Loma Linda, CA.

HURD, FRANK J. D.C. and ROSALIE HURD B.S., *The Ten Talents,* The College Press, Collegedale, TN.

GREGORY, DICK; *Natural Diet for Folks Who Eat: Cookin' with Mother Nature.* Harper & Row.

ROYAL, PENNY C.; *Herbally Yours,* Sound Nutrition, Provo, UT.

MALSTROM, STAN; N.D., M.T., *Own Your Own Body,* Woodland Books, UT.

TENNEY, LOUISE; *Todays Herbal Health,* Woodland Books, UT.

WALKER, NORMAN W. D.S.C., Ph.D; *Colon Health: The Key to a Vibrant Life,* Norwalk Press, Prescott, Arizona.

ROBBINS, JOHN; *Diet for a New America*, Stillpoint Publishing, Walpole, N.H.

GRAY, HENRY F.R.S; *Gray's Anatomy* , Running Press, Philadelphia, PA.

KLOSS , JETHRO and Family; *The Back to Eden Cookbook*, Back to Eden Books, Loma Linda, CA.

POLUNIN, MIRIAM; *Minerals*, Thorsons Publishers, New York,

HONOR, IDA of E. MCBEAN, *Vaccination: The Silent Killer,* Honor Publications, Cutten, CA.

LIDELL, LUCINDA; *The Book of Massage,* Simon & Shuster.

WEED ASH, SUSAN; *Wise Woman Herbal for the Childbearing Year,* Tree Publishing; Woodstock, NY.

BROOKS, KAREN; *The Complete Vegetarian Cookbook,* Simon & Shuster.

NOSS WHITNEY, ELEANOR and EVA MAY Nunnelley; *Understanding Nutrition* Hamilton, West Publishing, NY

ADAMS, REX; *Miracle Medicine Foods,* Warner Books, NY

WALKER, N.W., D. SCIENCE, *Raw Vegetable Juices,* Jove Books, 200 Madison Avenue, NY

SHURTLEFF, WILLIAM and AKIKO AOYAGI; *The Book of Tofu,* Ballantine Books, NY

ABAYOMI, GYASI; *Natural Cures for the Body,* Alkebulan Academy Press, PA.

KULBINSKAS, VIKTORAS; *Survival into the 21st Century,* Woodstock Valley, CT.

TENNEY, LOUISE; *Today's Healthy Eating,* Woodland Books, Provo, UT.

HON. ELIJAH MUHAMMAD; *How to Eat to Live: Book 1,* Muhammad's Temple of Islam Chicago,

ELLIOT, ROSE; *Vegetarian Mother Baby Book,* Pantheon Books, NY.

DIAMOND, HARVEY and MARILYN; *Fit for Life ,* Warner Books, NY.

CLAESSENS, SHARON; *The 20-Minute Foods Cookbook,* Rodale Press, Emmaus, PA.

DUFTY, WILLIAM; *The Sugar Blues ,*Warner Books, NY.

YUDKIN, JOHN M.D; *Sweet and Dangerouss,* Bantam Books, NY.

Magazines

New Frontier Magazine, 421 Fairmont Avenue, Philadelphia, PA 19123.

Delicious Magazine, New Hope Communications, 328 South Main Street, New Hope, PA. 18938.

Let's Live Magazine, P. O. Box 749008, Los Angeles, CA. 90004.

Vegetarian Times, P. O. Box 570, Oak Park, IL. 60303.

Bestways Magazine, P. O. Box 570, Oak Park, IL. 60303.

Visions, 2531 Huntingdon Pike, Huntingdon Valley, PA. 19006.

East West Journal, Kushi Foundation, Inc., 17 Station Street, Box 1200, Brookline, MA. 02147.

Health Federation Magazine, National Health Federation, 212 W. Foodhill, P. O. Box 688, Monrovia,CA. 91016.

Earth Save, 706 Frederick Street, Santa Cruz, CA 95062-2205

ILLUSTRATION OF COLON

A healthy normal size colon

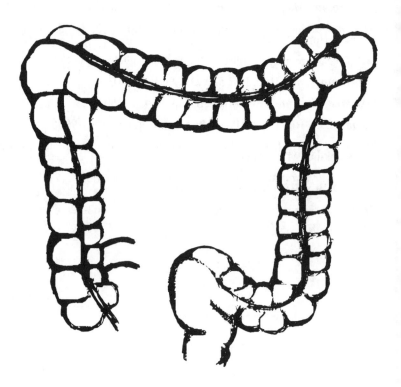

The colon is an extremely important determinant of body health. If we eat improperly the shape and size of the colon can be perverted and distorted. An unhealthy colon is the root cause of the majority of health problems.

ILLUSTRATION OF HERB ECHINACEA

The Herb Echinacea

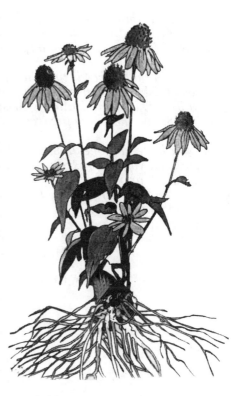

BOTANICAL NAME:
Echinacea Angustifolia
COMMON NAME:
Echinacea, the Sampson root
and the purple coneflower.
PART USED : ROOTS

DESCRIPTION

Flowers: Composite flower
head, solitary, 3-4 inches
across; cone shaped center
composed of numerous tiny,
purple and tubular florets;
surrounded by 15 - 20
spreading purple ray florets.
Leaves. Pale green to dark
green; lower leaves are
pointed, ovate, coarsely
tooted and 3-8 in. long;
upper leaves shorter and
narrower.
Height: Grows 1-2 ft.

Echinacea is one of the most powerful herbs in the herb kingdom. It
is very effective in alleviating mucous, colds, flu, sore throat, tonsillitis, high cholesterol, cancer, boils, swellings, infections, childhood
diseases, skin problems, inflammations, insect bites impure blood,
blood poisoning, and sexually transmitted diseases. It is also an excellent enhancer for the immune system.

FINAL COMMENT

I'd like to thank you for purchasing this book. I trust that you found it beneficial. Please purchase as many books as you desire for friends, relatives and special gifts.

A part of the proceeds that this writing generates will go toward establishing a non-profit community self-improvement organization. This organization will seek to enhance individual self-esteem and aid in conflict resolution.

If you have any questions about herbs, nutrition, or health you can send your correspondence to the below address. If you would like to order herbs or would like a response to your inquiry, please include a self-addressed, stamped envelop and your telephone number.

Keith T. Wright
Health Masters
P. O. Box 28003
Philadelphia, PA 19131

INDEX

A&B Publishers Group
SELECTED TITLES

A BOOK OF THE BEGINNINGS VOL. I & II	40.00
AFRIKAN HOLISTIC HEALTH	15.95
AFRICAN DISCOVERY OF AMERICA	10.00
A HEALTHY FOODS AND SPIRITUAL NUTRITION HANDBOOK	8.95
ARAB INVASION OF EGYPT & THE FIRST 30 YEARS OF ROMAN DOMINION	14.95
ANACALYPSIS (SET)	40.00
ANACALYPSIS VOL. 1	25.00
ANACALYPSIS VOL. 11	20.00
AIDS THE END OF CIVILIZATION	9.95
CHRISTOPHER COLUMBUS & THE AFRICAN HOLOCAUST	10.00
COLUMBUS CONSPIRACY	11.95
DAWN VOYAGE:THE BLACK AFRICAN DISCOVERY OF AMERICA	11.95
EDUCATION OF THE NEGRO	9.95
EGYPTIAN BOOK OF THE DEAD . . . . E. W. BUDGE	9.95
EGYPTIAN BOOK OF THE DEAD/ANCIENT MYSTERIES OF AMENTA G. MASSEY	9.95
EVERYTHING YOU NEEDED TO KNOW ABOUT HAIRLOCKING	7.95
FIRST COUNCIL OF NICE	9.95
GOSPEL OF BARNABAS	8.95
GERALD MASSEY'S LECTURES	9.95
GLOBAL AFRIKAN PRESENCE	14.95
HARLEM VOICES	11.95
HARLEM USA	11.95
HEAL THYSELF FOR HEALTH AND LONGEVITY	9.95
HEAL THYSELF COOKBOOK:HOLISTIC COOKING WITH JUICES	9.95
HISTORICAL JESUS & THE MYTHICAL CHRIST	9.95
LOST BOOKS OF THE BIBLE & THE FORGOTTEN BOOKS OF EDEN	9.95
RAPE OF PARADISE	14.95
SIGNS & SYMBOLS OF PRIMORDIAL MAN	16.95
THE TWO BABYLONS (666 THE MARK OF THE BEAST REVEALED)	14.95
VACCINES ARE DANGEROUS: A WARNING TO THE BLACK COMMUNITY	9.95
VITAMINS & MINERALS FROM A TO Z	9.95
FREEMASONRY INTERPRETED	12.95
FREEMASONRY & THE VATICAN	9.95
FREEMASONRY & JUDAISM	9.95
FREEMASONRY:CHARACTER & CLAIMS	9.95
SECRET SOCIETY	11.95
FREEMASONRY EXPOSITION: EXPOSITION & ILLUSTRATIONS OF FREEMASONRY	9.95

Send for our complete catalog now!

Mail To:**A&B PUBLISHERS GROUP · 1000 ATLANTIC AVE · NEW YORK · 11238**

TEL: (718)783-7808 · FAX (718)783-7267

Name:_____

Address_____

City_____ST_____Zip_____

Card Type_____Card Number_____

Exp____/_____ *Signature* _____

We accept VISA MASTERCARD AMERICAN EXPRESS & DISCOVER